IMAGES
of America

BAYSTATE FRANKLIN MEDICAL CENTER

HOSPITAL RATES.

Open Ward, per day - - - - $1.50
Two Bed Room, per day - - - $2.00
Private Room, per day - $2.50, $3.00 and $4.00

SPECIAL NURSE

From Training School - $17.50 per week
From Outside of Hospital $25.00 per week
Board for special nurse $5.00 per week.

Fee for Use of Operating Room or Maternity Room $5.00

Meals (for visitors)

Breakfast 25 cts. Dinner 50 cts. Supper 25 cts.

The hours for visiting are 2.00 to 4.00 and 7.00 to 8.00 P. M. If visitors desire admission at other hours, permission must be obtained from the superintendent or the head nurse.

Stationery, postal cards, postage stamps and tooth brushes may be obtained upon request.

For excessive dressings and certain special medical and surgical supplies, special prices are charged, depending upon their cost.

For radiographs, special laboratory examinations, etc., special arrangements must be made.

The rate for this room is $3.00 per day.

Shown is a copy of Franklin County Public Hospital's rate card from 1903. Open ward beds cost $1.50, semi-private rooms $2, and private rooms up to $4. Special nurses were extra, with lower rates for nurses in training. Use of the delivery or operating rooms cost $5 extra. Visiting hours were from 2:00 to 4:00 p.m. and 7:00 to 8:00 p.m., unless special permission was obtained from the head nurse. (Courtesy of Baystate Franklin Medical Center.)

On the Cover: Franklin County Public Hospital occupied converted houses prior to construction of dedicated hospital facilities on High Street in 1910. This 1903 photograph shows nurses at work at the second-floor nursing station. The hospital occupied the former private residence of James Converse between 1898 and 1910. (Courtesy of Baystate Franklin Medical Center.)

IMAGES
of America

Baystate Franklin Medical Center

Thomas L. Higgins, MD, Sandra W. Campbell,
and Gina O. Campbell, RN

ARCADIA
PUBLISHING

ISBN 978-1-4671-1701-2

Published by Arcadia Publishing
Charleston, South Carolina

Printed in the United States of America

Library of Congress Control Number: 2016938431

For all general information, please contact Arcadia Publishing:
Telephone 843-853-2070
Fax 843-853-0044
E-mail sales@arcadiapublishing.com
For customer service and orders:
Toll-Free 1-888-313-2665

Visit us on the Internet at www.arcadiapublishing.com

To the physicians, nurses, and all team members who have fulfilled the promise of "keeping care local" espoused by the citizens of Franklin County in 1895. To our spouses and children, in appreciation for their support of our endeavors, both clinical and historical. To all who came before us and to those who will follow in the mission of improving the health of our community every day.

Contents

ACKNOWLEDGMENTS

We would like to thank Baystate Franklin Medical Center (BFMC) and the many people and departments that contributed to this project. We are especially indebted to Phyllis Stone at BFMC for her knowledge of Franklin County Public Hospital (FCPH) history, and to Greg Oles for his comprehensive knowledge of buildings and dates. Background information for photographs was graciously provided by the Pioneer Valley Museum Association, Historic Deerfield, Deerfield Academy, Northfield Historical Society, the *Greenfield Recorder*, and Lyndley Wilson at the Greenfield Historical Society. Photograph captions were also augmented with reference to previously published sources, especially *The Conservative Rebel* by Paul Jenkins, published in 1982. Other important sources were annual reports of Franklin County Public Hospital, brochures from the FCPH School of Nursing, records of the Baystate Franklin Auxiliary (previously the Board of Organized Work) and archives of the Birthplace at BFMC. We would like to thank the many past and present FCPH and BFMC employees who shared their recollections, as well as members of the Baystate Franklin Auxiliary.

Unless otherwise noted, images in this volume were drawn from the archives of BFMC; others are credited to the Pocumtuck Valley Memorial Association (PVMA), Greenfield Historical Society (GHS), Historic Deerfield (HD), Deerfield Academy (DA), Northfield Historical Society (NHS), and the *Greenfield Recorder* (GR). Items from the authors' personal collections are credited as TLH, SWC, or GOC. We also appreciate the help of Maggie Humberston at the Lyman & Merrie Wood Museum of Springfield History, which houses the archives of Springfield Hospital/ Baystate Medical Center and Baystate Health. Jodi Olmsted, Todd Lajoie, and Kent Spiry were instrumental in scanning photographs and artwork from the various sources. Special thanks go to Suzanne Hendery, vice president of marketing and public affairs, who facilitated this project. In addition, we would like to acknowledge Jim Bassett, Mary and Bruce Mainville, and Judy Fusonie for their assistance in the final proofing of this book.

INTRODUCTION

The spirit of today's mission for Baystate Franklin Medical Center—to improve the health of its community—can be traced back to 1894, when Greenfield and Franklin County had no hospital. That year, Dr. Willard Pierce, assisted by Ellen Brown of Leyden, rented a house at 6 Main Street, opening a private hospital to demonstrate the community need. Shortly after, prominent citizen Dr. Adams Calhoun Deane advocated establishing a public hospital, rallying the community to this cause. On March 2, 1895, thirty-six citizens of Franklin County signed an agreement to establish the Franklin County Public Hospital. Together with the people of Greenfield and the surrounding communities of Shelburne, Shelburne Falls, Colrain, Leyden, Bernardston, Northfield, Gill, Turners Falls, Millers Falls, Montague, Deerfield, and Conway, a vision was forged, with over $16,000 raised during the initial fundraising campaign. The hospital opened on September 9, 1895, in the former home of the Reverend Dr. Francis Robbins, a prominent local minister who later founded the Robbins Memorial Church. Fifty-five patients were served the first year, with an annual operating budget of just under $6,000. The fledgling hospital was also fortunate to receive substantial donations from former Franklin County residents, including $10,000 from Maria Luthera Hovey Hosmer (1829–1923) of Brooklyn, New York, the daughter of physician Daniel Hovey (1782–1874) of Greenfield.

Growth was swift. In 1898, the board of managers voted to purchase the Converse property at the corner of Main and Conway Streets for the sum of $13,000. This purchase was funded in large part by the gift of $10,000 by Greenfield native Judge Charles Allen, now of Boston. By 1901, limitations of the existing facilities were apparent, and plans were already underway to build a new hospital on empty land on High Street. In 1906, a building committee was established, led by Dr. H.G. Stetson, F.A. Pond, and J.D. Kiley, aiming for an ambitious fundraising goal of $50,000. The Honorable Levi J. Gunn helped kick off the campaign with a gift of $10,000, and land was purchased at the corner of High and Beacon Streets, augmented by a gift of contiguous land by Mrs. John Sheldon and Mrs. George Sheldon. Plans were drawn up by the Boston architectural firm Kendall, Taylor & Stevens. By 1910, when the South and Administration Buildings were opened, over $65,000 in money and pledges had been received. In addition, local physicians Drs. Twitchell, Stetson, and Canedy provided and installed X-ray equipment. Levi Gunn served as president from the hospital's inception until he stepped down in October 1914. His successor, E.B. Blake, served as president until March 1917, succeeded by Dr. Halbert G. Stetson. The hospital was seriously challenged by the 1918 influenza pandemic. During a six-week period in September and October of that year, 135 patients were admitted, with 46 deaths. Porches were hastily converted to patient wards, and one outcome of the epidemic was the construction and opening of a nearby isolation hospital funded by the Town of Greenfield.

Childbirth was not always a hospital event; in the 1800s, hospitalization was generally avoided by those with resources to deliver at home with or without the assistance of a midwife. When Franklin County Public Hospital was established, the vast majority of births still took place at home, despite sanitary advances that had by then reduced the incidence of puerperal (childbed) fever. Caesarian sections were introduced in 1894, X-rays in 1895, and "twilight sleep" to ease the pain of labor in 1914, and gradually in-hospital obstetric care became a symbol of progress. In much of the industrialized world, childbirth became a medical procedure by the 1950s. Only later did the pendulum begin to swing back, with new appreciation for midwives and birthing centers, with FCPH pioneering these changes. Water births were inaugurated at FCPH in 1980. The Birthing Center, led by nurse manager Dorothy Telega, offered private suites, water birth tubs, and Jacuzzi-style whirlpools in an environment where high-risk obstetric and surgical care could still be provided when necessary.

Education of nurses formed an important part of the hospital's function right from the start. The first group of nurses educated at FCPH graduated in September 1897, and annual graduations followed thereafter until nursing education was transferred to Greenfield Community College in the fall of 1965. Initially, the nurses lived and worked in the hospital itself, occupying the top floors in the converted houses. Between 1915 and 1927, student nurses lived at a house (still standing today) at the corner of High and Beacon Streets. Students provided much of the care delivered to patients, under the supervision of a small staff of hospital-employed nurses. Nellie Daniels was the first superintendent of nurses, from 1895 to 1896, followed by Annie C. Nedwell (1897–1900), Mrs. M.H. Lawrence (1901), Anna M. Sweeney (1901–1917) and Annie S. Barclay (1918–1950).

The Women's Board of Organized Work (originally called the Organized Work Committee) was created in 1895 and became one of the hospital's principal benefactors. It was the ninth hospital auxiliary to be established in Massachusetts. The founding members were Mrs. A.C. Deane (chairwoman), Julia Ulrich, Mrs. F.R. Allen, Mrs. Emil Weissbrod, Mrs. L.A. Cook, Mrs. J.H. Sanderson, Mrs. Robert Abercrombie, Mrs. Henry E. Goodell, and Mary Ranahan. Over the years, and through its various incarnations as the Board of Organized Work (BOOW) and now the Baystate Franklin Auxiliary (BFA), volunteers have undertaken projects generating many thousands of dollars and contributed substantially to the stability and welfare of the hospital. In 1900, a "free bed" was established, which permitted any person in Franklin County to receive free nursing care and medical attention as recommended by a physician. Sunshine Boxes were introduced in 1921 to collect coins for nursing scholarships. Funds were also raised by sales of home-canned food, whist parties, charity balls, lawn parties, and cookbooks first published in 1937. In 1951, the BOOW established the hospital's gift shop, which today remains one of the most successful fundraising endeavors and a favorite place to shop for staff and visitors alike. From 1965 to the 1990s, the Junior Branch of the BOOW operated a coffee shop with the idea that younger volunteers could pay their dues and then graduate to full membership in the BOOW. Over the years, the BOOW supported the student volunteers (candy stripers) and ran a beauty shop within the hospital called the Head Shed. Today, the BFA remains a major contributor to the hospital.

In the 50 years from the hospital's founding to 1945, some 50,649 patient records had been created, each reflecting at least one hospital admission. Many thousands more were seen in outpatient settings. The Cancer Clinic, a progressive collaboration with the rival Farren Memorial Hospital, was established in 1928, and sessions alternated each month between locations. The Children's Clinic under Dr. Merritt B. Low and the Heart Clinic under Dr. Harriet Hardy were established in 1937. In those days, health care was largely delivered by local general practitioners (GPs) who would refer to local surgeons and specialists. Each GP or surgeon would admit and care for his or her own patients when hospitalization was necessary. During the Depression years of the 1930s, hospitalization insurance had gained wide acceptance, and FCPH was one of the first institutions to accept the plan of the Hospital Service Corporation, now known as Blue Cross/Blue Shield. Employer-paid health insurance became an enticing employee benefit when wage controls were imposed during World War II. Many hospitals, including FCPH, had struggled financially during the 1930s. In the early postwar years, more widespread insurance benefits, medical advances derived from increased research funding, and the prosperity that helped create the Baby Boom ushered in a golden era for hospital growth. After the war, the hospital began to recruit new specialists, including fulltime pathologist Aaron W. Newton, radiologist Donald P. Hamm, and anesthesiologist Philip D. Woodbridge.

In August 1962, the FCPH building committee was tasked to design new hospital facilities. A development committee chaired by Channing L. Bete, Joseph W. Ballard Jr., and Walker J. Hosmer worked with more than 100 citizens, deciding on a $2.5-million expansion project to provide 72 new hospital beds. Over the next four years, the building committee consulted with physicians, nurses, hospital employees, patients, architects, and hospital consultants regarding various design proposals. Ultimately, the committee accepted the recommendations of director Bright M. Dornblaster and architect Sherman Morss to proceed with the "spoke design," a concept previously not seen in hospital design. The three-spoke project (now Spokes II-IV) began in August 1966 and was completed in February 1968. The East Spoke (now Spoke I, housing the Mental Health Unit) was begun in April 1968 and was finished in September 1969. The final West Spoke (now Spoke V) was started in December 1968 and was completed in July 1970. The entire project cost more than $5 million, including relocation of other key services.

The Medicare program was enacted in 1965, followed by provision of Medicaid assistance to the nation's poorest families. The Social Security Amendments of 1972 extended Medicare beyond the elderly to those with end-stage renal disease or severe disability. With millions more now covered by health insurance funded by payroll taxes, health care services again expanded, and most hospitals saw dramatic increases in patient volume. Telemetry technology originally developed for the NASA space program found its way to hospitals, which were establishing coronary care and intensive care units. Improvements in medical and surgical techniques provided new treatment options, and longevity began to increase. Franklin County Public Hospital continued to grow and again desperately needed new surgical capacity, including facilities to permit patients having minor surgery to have "day surgery," an emerging concept at the time. The Russell Surgical Building was opened in 1975.

FCPH's affiliation with Baystate Medical Center (BMC) in Springfield began in 1981, initially with a cooperative agreement to share clinical, laboratory, library, and medical education resources. In 1983, FCPH was renamed Franklin Medical Center (FMC), and in 1986, BMC and FMC joined to create Baystate Health Systems, with 3,822 employees and an $87-million payroll. Since then, Baystate Health has grown to become the premier integrated health network in Western Massachusetts, with over 12,000 employees. Baystate Health today includes Baystate Medical Center in Springfield (incorporating the former Springfield and Wesson Hospitals), BFMC, Baystate Mary Lane Hospital in Ware, Baystate Wing Hospital in Palmer, Baystate Noble Hospital in Westfield, Baystate Medical Practices, the Baystate Visiting Nurses Association, and the Health New England insurance company. Despite the challenges of financing health care in 2016, the future looks bright for BFMC as part of a large, stable, integrated system.

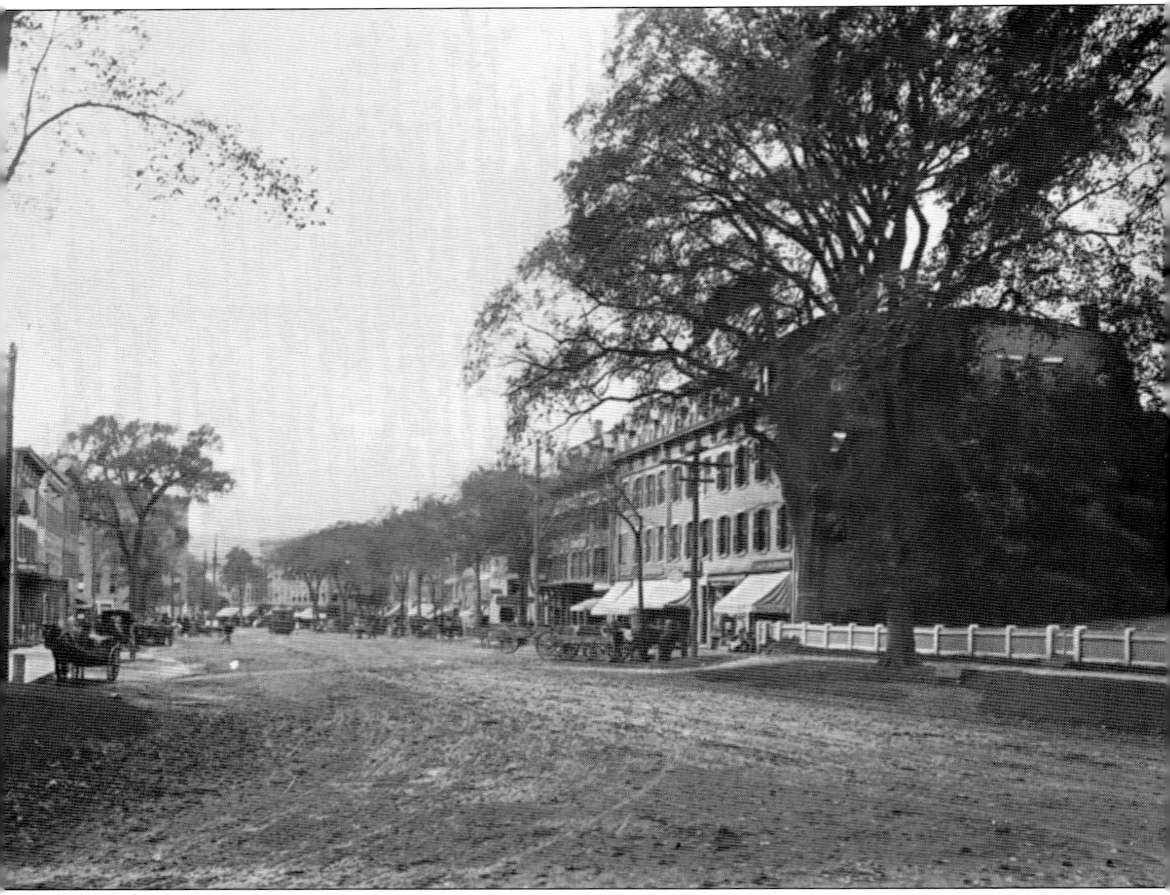

Greenfield, Massachusetts, is pictured around 1890. The town sits in a broad, shallow valley defined by the Shelburne hills to the west, the Leyden hills to the north, and the Rocky Mountain ridge, which tracks the Connecticut River to the east. Native Americans of the Pocumtuck tribe settled the region some 11,000 years ago following the retreat of glacial ice sheets. European settlement dates to 1686, and the town was incorporated in 1753, carved from neighboring Deerfield. By 1890, the town had a population of 5,252 and was thriving on the manufacture of taps and dies, cutlery, and machinery. (Courtesy of Peter Miller.)

One

FCPH IN THE 19TH CENTURY

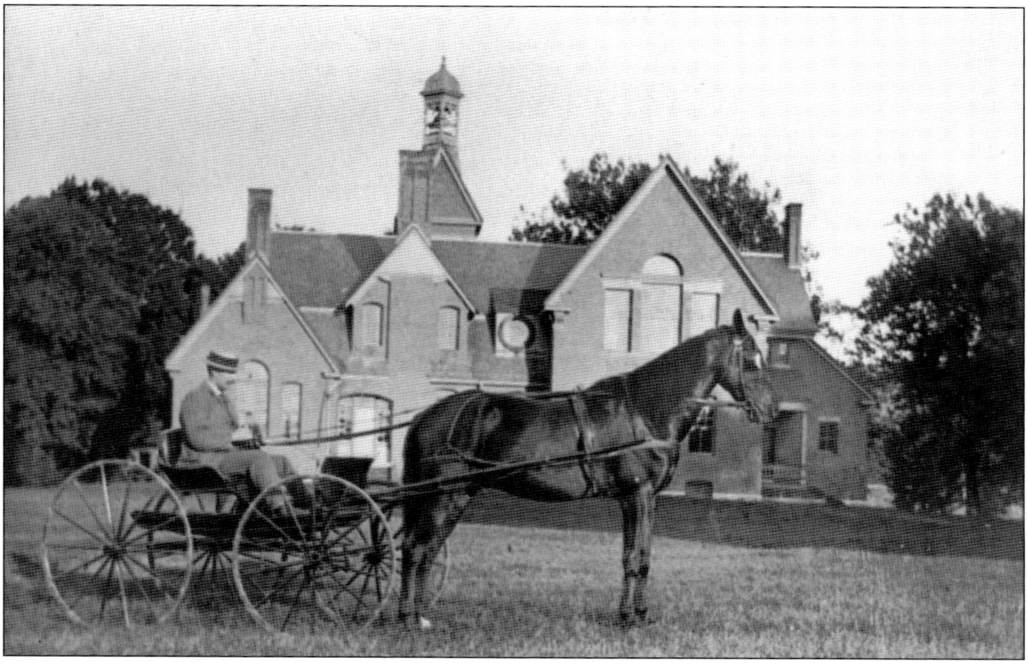

Dr. Franklin Spilman Newell (1854–1895) is shown in his horse-drawn buggy with the Deerfield Academy/Dickinson High School building behind him. Dr. Newell was a native of Readsboro, Vermont, and a graduate of the University of Vermont's Medical College. He practiced in Deerfield from 1886 until a tragic accident in 1895. He died shortly after being thrown from a horse-drawn sleigh while visiting a patient. In the era before automobiles, physicians traveled to patients' homes via foot, bicycle, or horse. The Franklin District Medical Society was established in Greenfield in 1851; the founding officers were Stephen W. Williams, James Deane, and Alpheus Stone. By 1880, at least 67 physicians were practicing in Franklin County. (PVMA.)

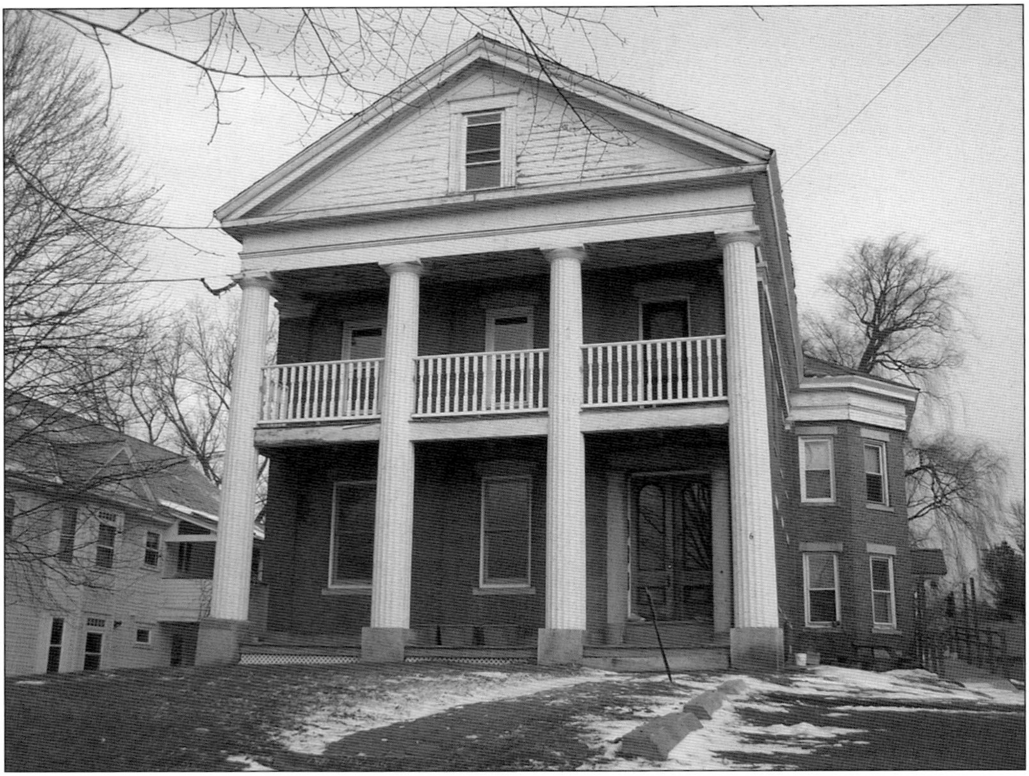

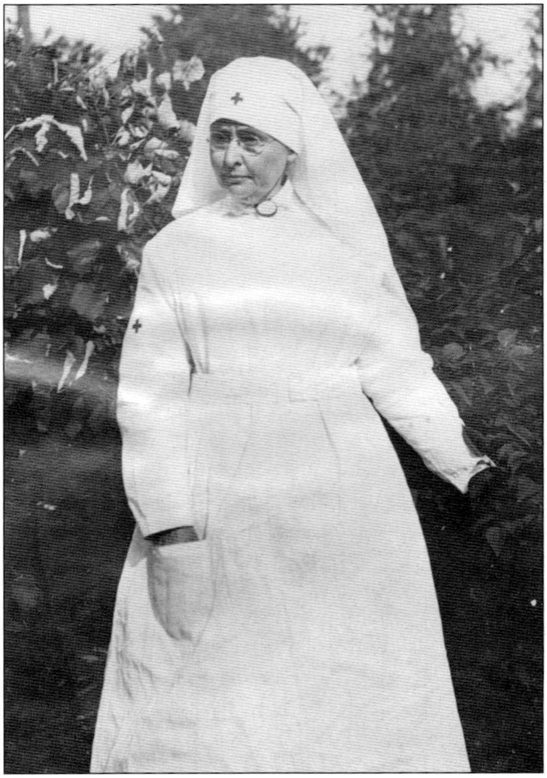

Dr. Willard Pierce, a local physician, rented this house at 6 Main Street in September 1894, operating it as a private hospital to demonstrate the growing need in the community for care that could not be adequately provided in a home. Once it was determined that the Franklin County Public Hospital would be opening in September 1895, Dr. Pierce closed his private hospital in July 1895 and merged with FCPH. The columned brick house (pictured) still stands today. Ellen Leisring Brown, daughter of Samuel Childs Brown and Sarah Anne McCloud Brown of Leyden, was the first nurse assisting Dr. Pierce. (TLH.)

Ellen L. Brown (1863–1959) graduated from the nursing school at Massachusetts General Hospital in 1890 and encouraged Dr. Willard Pierce to establish his private hospital in 1894, where she became head nurse. In this 1944 photograph, she was still working at the Red Cross Center in Greenfield at the age of 81. She lived to the age of 96.

Dr. Adams Calhoun Deane (1823–1899) was a native of Colrain, a surgeon, and the son, nephew, and grandson of locally prominent physicians. Deane studied at Deerfield Academy and received his medical doctorate from the University of New York in 1849. After medical school, he entered practice with his father in Colrain, served as a member of the General Court of Massachusetts, and helped organize the Franklin County Medical Society. When his uncle, Dr. James Deane of Greenfield, passed away in 1858, Adams took over his thriving practice. Deane was considered the founding father of Franklin County Public Hospital, having advocated its establishment by 1894, and engineering an agreement of association signed by 36 citizens on March 2, 1895. The community raised over $16,000 during the first fundraising campaign by holding a fair. Dr. Deane died at the age of 76 on November 7, 1899. (GHS.)

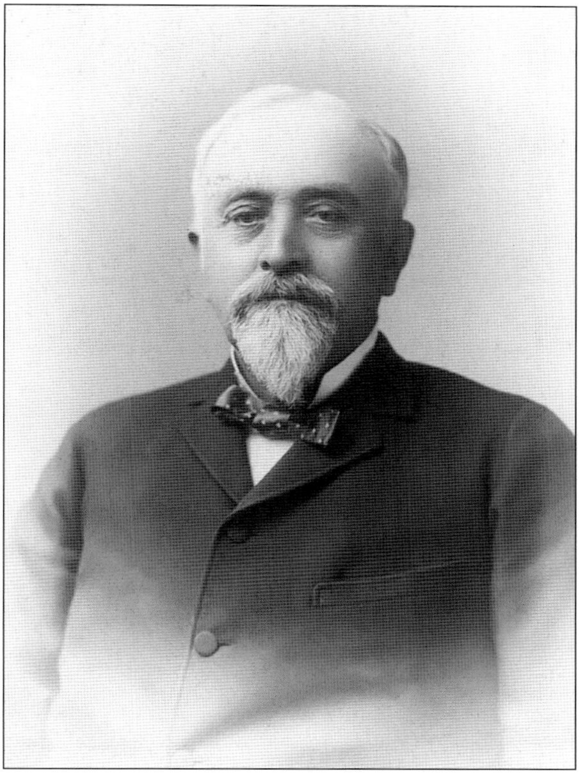

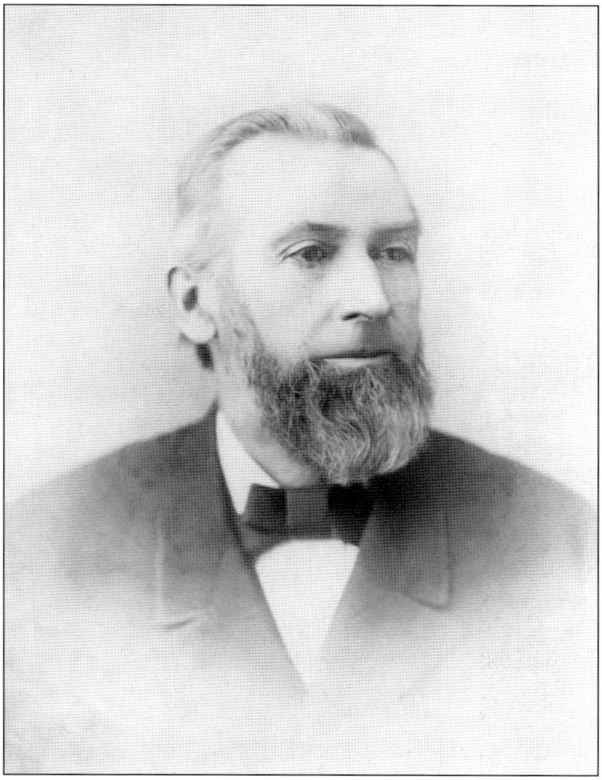

Levi J. Gunn (pictured) and Charles H. Amidon were in their early 30s when they founded Gunn and Amidon, a major producer of wringers to squeeze the water from freshly laundered clothes. In 1862, they received a patent for their Amidon Wringer, which was demonstrated at the New York State Fair and went on to sell over 20,000 units by 1863. Later, the company manufactured highly successful drill bit braces. Levi Gunn subsequently was a member of the Massachusetts Senate in 1886–1887 and a member of the Greenfield Board of Selectmen, and became FCPH's first president, a post he held for 18 years. He died on September 9, 1916, in Greenfield. (GHS)

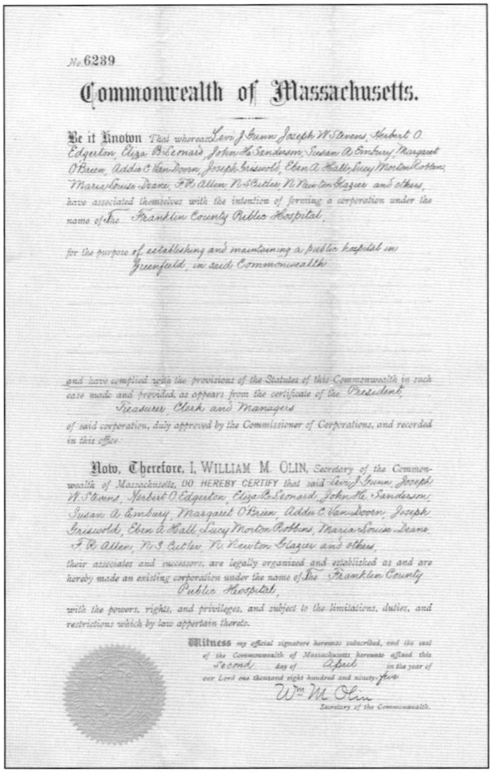

No. 6239

Commonwealth of Massachusetts.

Be it Known That whereas Levi J Gunn, Joseph W Stevens, Herbert O. Edgerton, Eliza B Leonard, John H Sanderson, Susan A Embury, Margaret O'Brien, Addie C VanDoorn, Joseph Griswold, Eben A Hall, Lucy Morton Robbins, Maria Louise Deane, F.R. Allen, N.S Cutler, N Newton Glazier and others, have associated themselves with the intention of forming a corporation under the name of The Franklin County Public Hospital,

for the purpose of establishing and maintaining a public hospital in Greenfield, in said Commonwealth

and have complied with the provisions of the Statutes of this Commonwealth in such case made and provided, as appears from the certificate of the President, Treasurer, Clerk and Managers of said corporation, duly approved by the Commissioner of Corporations, and recorded in this office:

Now, Therefore, I, WILLIAM M. OLIN, Secretary of the Commonwealth of Massachusetts, DO HEREBY CERTIFY that said Levi J Gunn, Joseph W. Stevens, Herbert O Edgerton, Eliza B Leonard, John H. Sanderson, Susan A Embury, Margaret O'Brien, Addie C VanDoorn, Joseph Griswold, Eben A Hall, Lucy Morton Robbins, Maria Louise Deane, F.R. Allen, N.S Cutler, N. Newton Glazier and others, their associates and successors, are legally organized and established as and are hereby made an existing corporation under the name of The Franklin County Public Hospital,

with the powers, rights, and privileges, and subject to the limitations, duties, and restrictions which by law appertain thereto.

Witness my official signature hereunto subscribed, and the seal of the Commonwealth of Massachusetts hereunto affixed this Second day of April in the year of our Lord one thousand eight hundred and ninety-five

Wm M Olin
Secretary of the Commonwealth.

The corporators of the hospital are listed on this document from April 2, 1895. They included Levi J. Gunn (president), Joseph W. Stevens (treasurer), Herbert O. Edgerton (secretary), Eliza B. Leonard, John H. Sanderson, Susan A. Embury, Margaret O'Brien, Addie C. VanDoorn, Joseph Griswold, Eben A. Hall, Lucy Morton Robbins, Maria Louise Deane, F.R. Allen, N.S. Cutler, N. Newton Glazier, "and others."

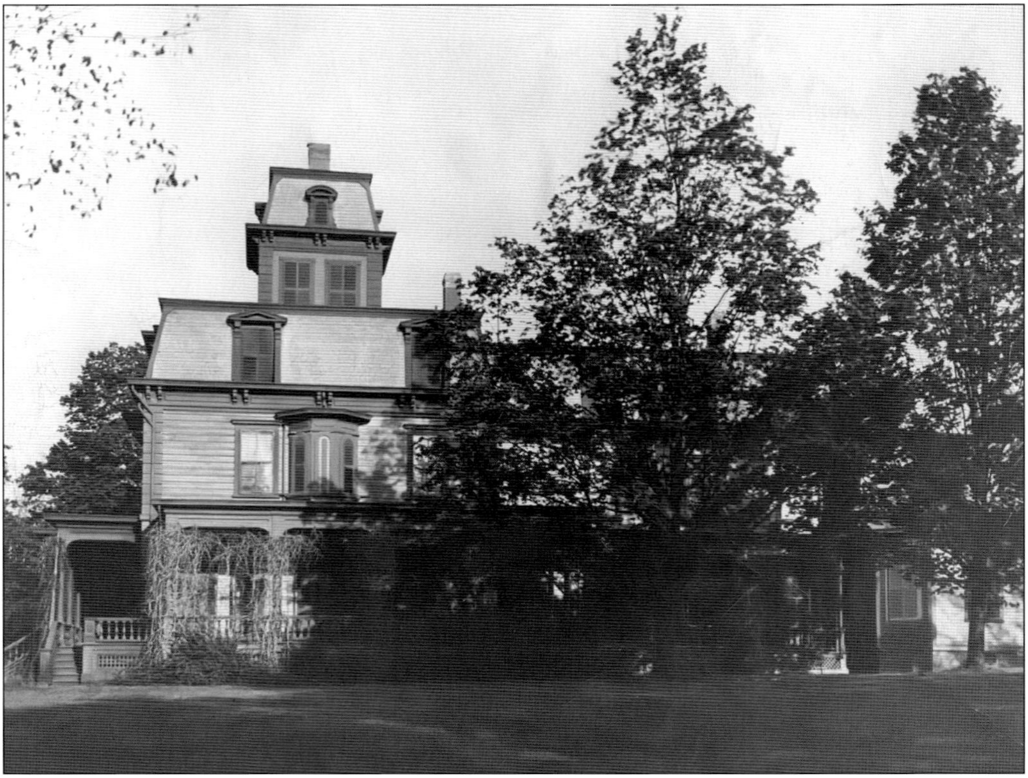

FCPH's first official home was on South Shelburne Road, just west of downtown Greenfield. The hospital opened on September 9, 1895, and served 55 patients in its first year with an annual budget of just under $6,000; the rent on the building was paid by local pledges. The hospital was an immediate success, with an average daily census of 10 to 15 patients treated at a cost of between $7 and $10 per week. All public patients were attended to and treated free of charge by members of the medical staff who happened to be on duty at that particular time. Within three years, FCPH would move to more spacious quarters.

The first Franklin County Public Hospital was housed in the former home of Rev. Dr. Francis L. Robbins, an Episcopal minister. The building was leased from Reverend Robbins for $1,000 per year. Nurses in training lived at the hospital. The Robbins Memorial Congregational Church was founded in 1892 and today occupies a building at 55 Munson Street, on the grounds of the original Robbins estate on South Shelburne Road. Coincidentally, Reverend Robbins was also the first patient admitted to the newly opened hospital. The building was razed in 1954.

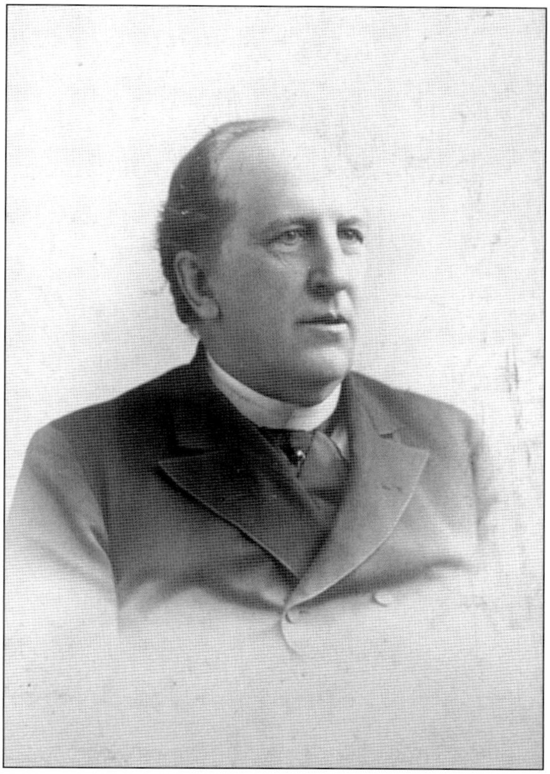

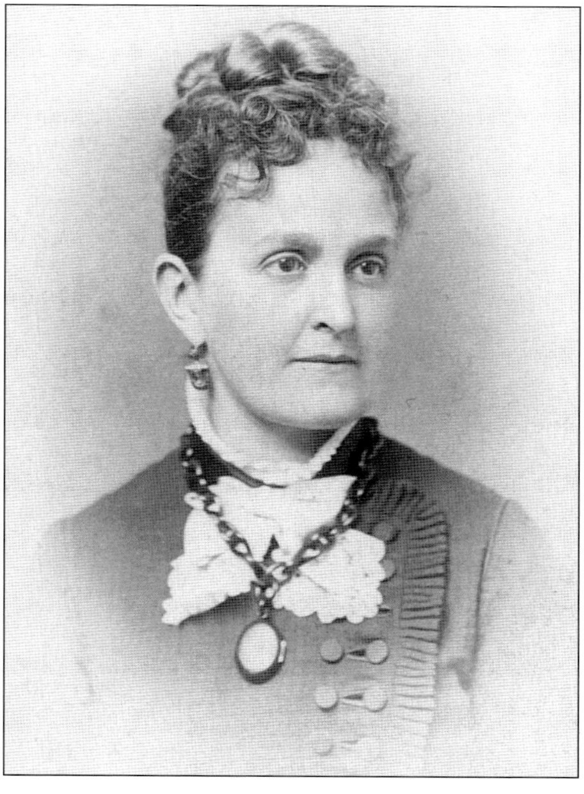

Maria Louise Grisold Deane was married to Dr. Adams Calhoun Dean and led the creation of the Women's Board of Organized Work. She was one of nine volunteers who formed one of the first hospital auxiliaries in Massachusetts in 1895. The BOOW worked on fundraising for the newly created hospital to meet unforeseen costs, and also did such tasks as sewing linens and collecting offerings of locally grown food for the patients' meals. (GHS.)

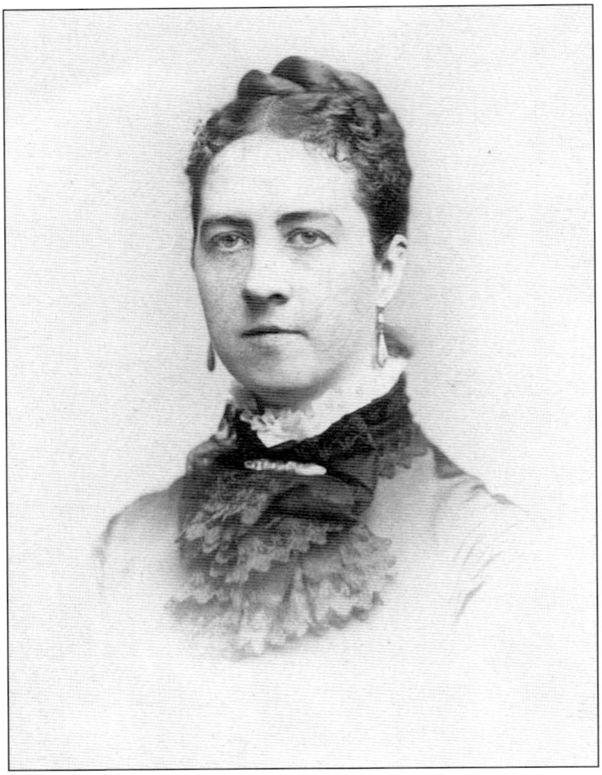

Eliza B. Leonard (1841–1933) was one of the original corporators of FCPH and an early benefactor and enthusiastic supporter of the hospital. In 1903, she was elected secretary to the hospital, the only woman to serve as an officer in the hospital's early years. Leonard donated to the hospital money she made selling homemade bread and cookies. A portrait of her by the artist H.S. Moskovitz was donated to FCPH by Alice N. Judd in 1963. Judd was at that time a member of the Board of Organized Work. The oil painting is now in the ownership of the Greenfield Historical Society as part of Greenfield's history. (GHS.)

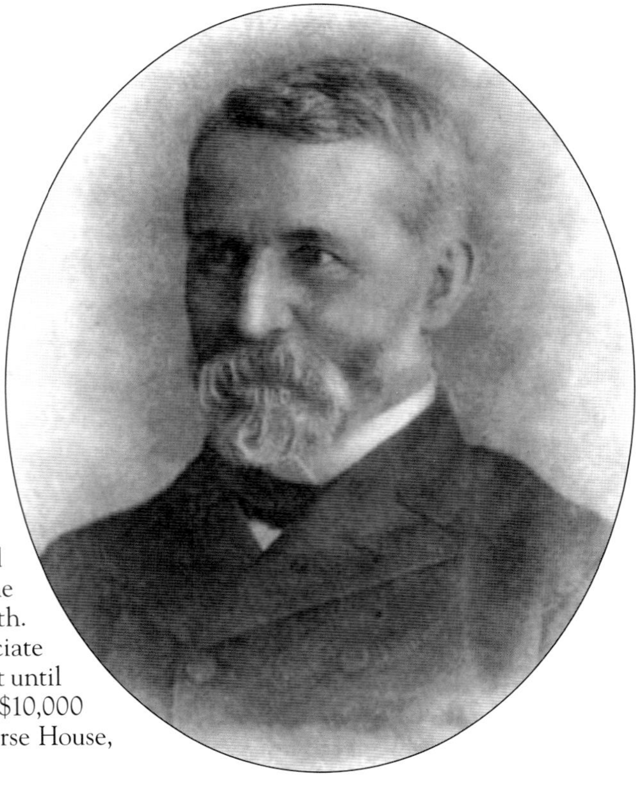

Judge Charles Allen (1827–1913) was born in Greenfield, graduated from Harvard College in 1847, and was admitted to the bar in Northampton in 1850. After practicing law for a dozen years in Greenfield, he advanced to state offices and was elected attorney general of Massachusetts in 1867, a post he held until 1872. Between 1880 and 1882, he chaired a commission whose work became the Public Statutes of the Commonwealth. He subsequently served as an associate justice of the Supreme Judicial Court until his retirement in 1898. His gift of $10,000 enabled the purchase of the Converse House, the second location of FCPH.

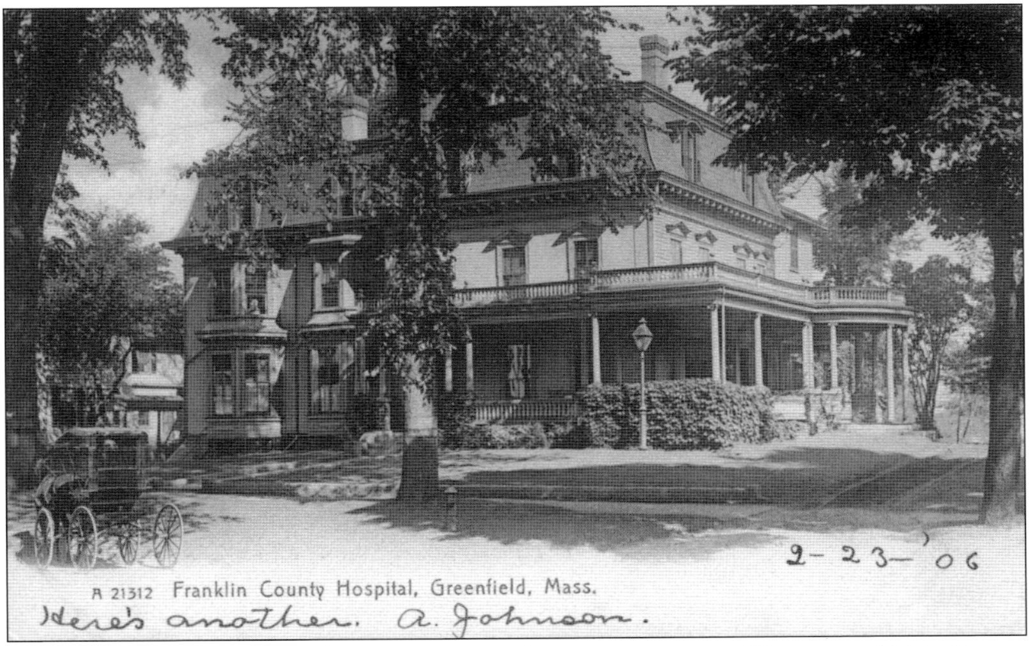

The second FCPH was located in the Converse House at the corner of Conway and Main Streets in Greenfield, which was rented from Henry Couillard in 1898. The once-elegant home was modified to include a state-of-the art operating room. However, the continued increase in patient volume drove the need to construct a bigger facility, and the Converse House was abandoned as a hospital in 1910.

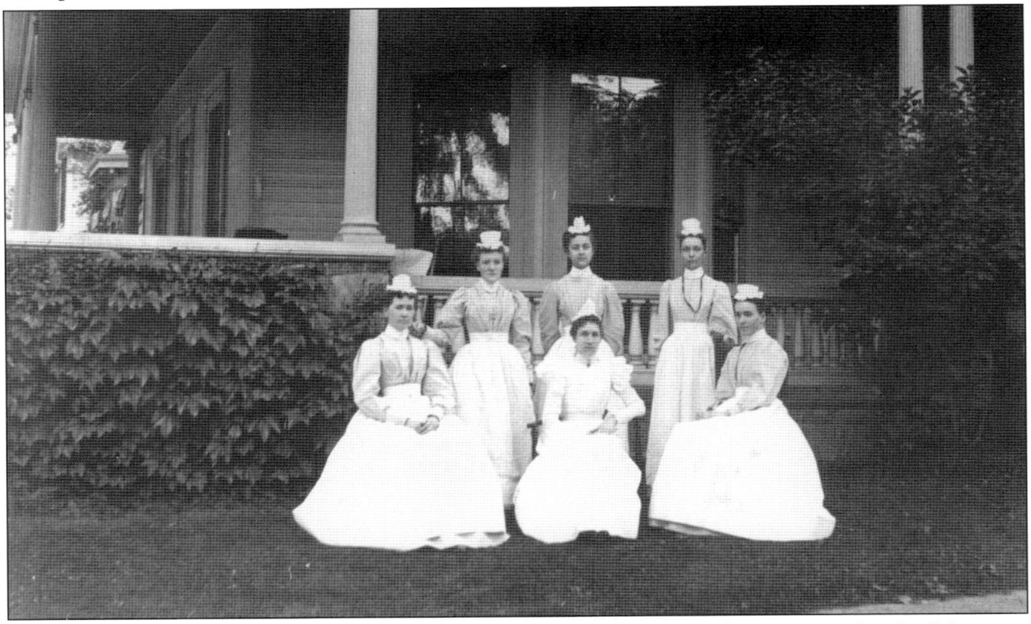

The nursing school class of 1898, the second class to graduate from the FCPH School of Nursing, is pictured here. From left to right are students Grace Page, Emily Young, Mrs. Field (who did not graduate), superintendent Katherine Martin (1897–1900), Annie C. Nedwell RN, and student Mary Conroy. They are shown outside the Converse House, which was the second location of the hospital from 1898 to 1910.

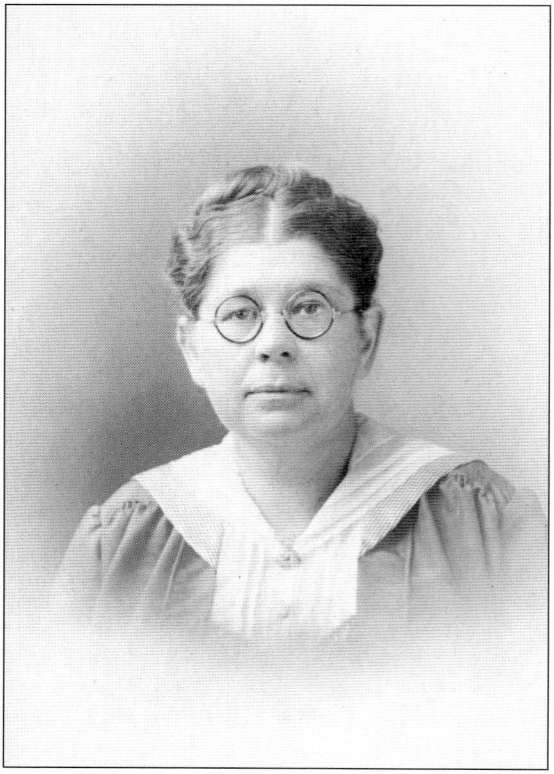

Clara Mary Greenough (1872–1963) was one of only two female physicians listed among the 17 physicians practicing in Greenfield in 1902. She attended Smith College and graduated from the Northwestern University Women's Medical School in 1899. Dr. Greenough worked in France and Germany during and after World War I and then returned to Greenfield in 1920. (PVMA.)

Nurses are preparing to dispense medications in this 1903 photograph. Note the "candlestick" telephone, the patient charts hanging from the wall, and the variety of medications in the cabinets. The stairway reflects the hospital's origin as a private home.

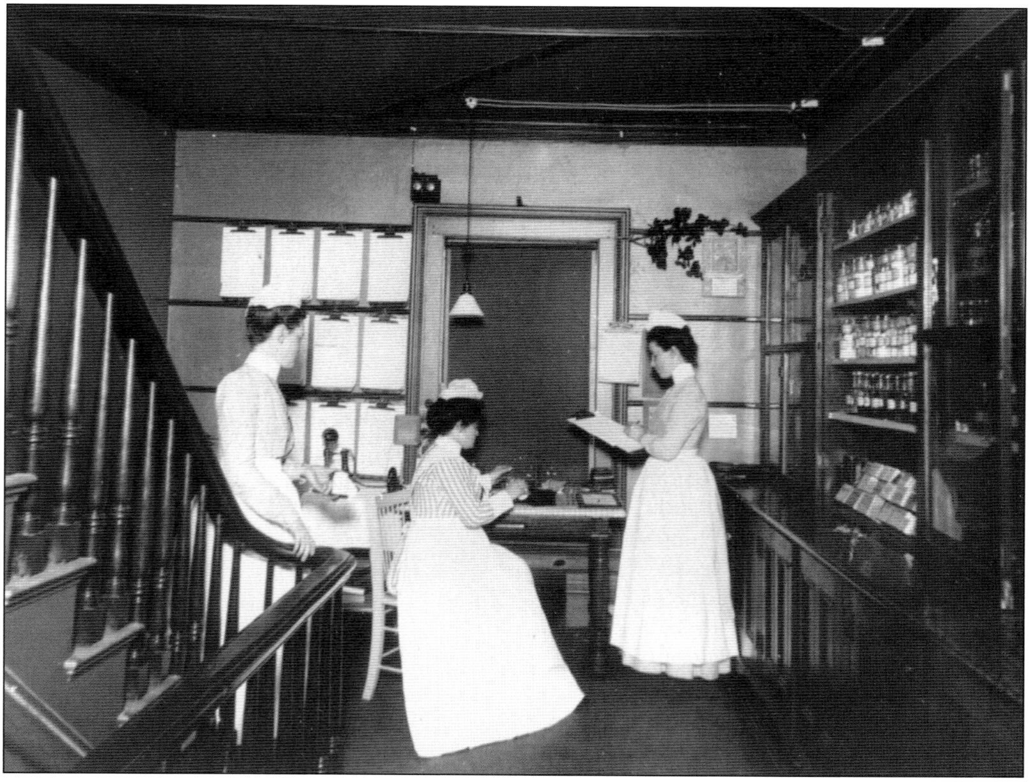

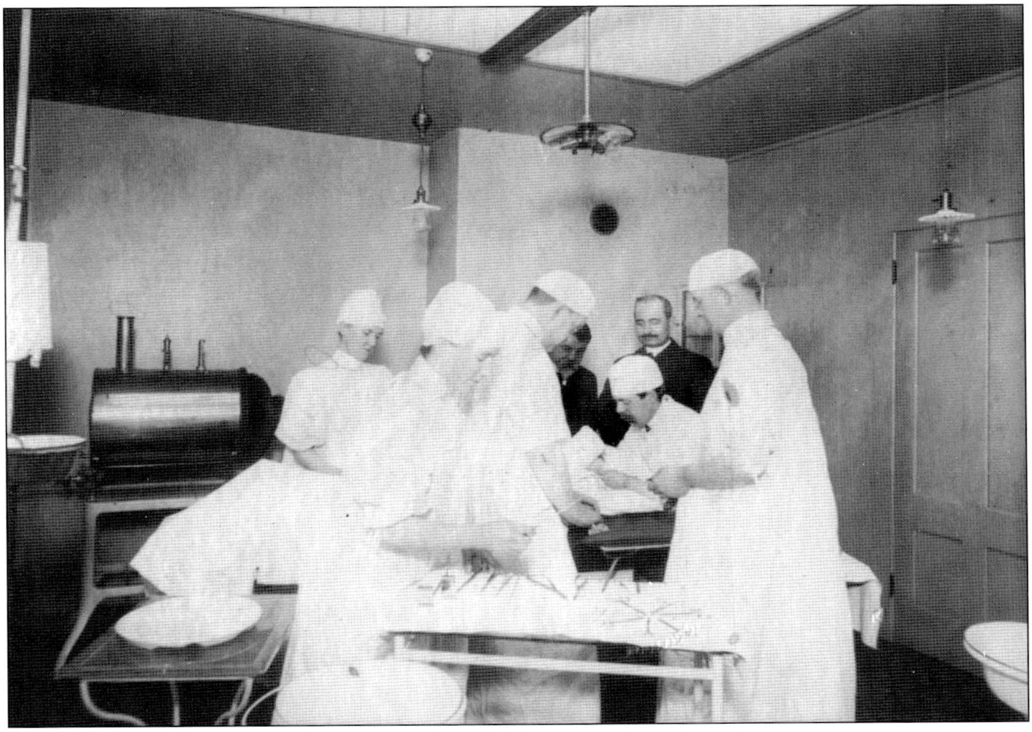

This 1903 photograph shows the operating room in the Converse House. From left to right are Nan Calhoun, Hester P. Millington (Gaines), Dr. Halbert G. Stetson, Dr. Enoch G. Best, Dr. Newton administering ether, Dr. Harry N. Howe, and Dr. Charles Canedy. As early as 1901, the limitations of this second hospital building were recognized, and plans were already being developed for a purpose-built hospital to be located on High Street.

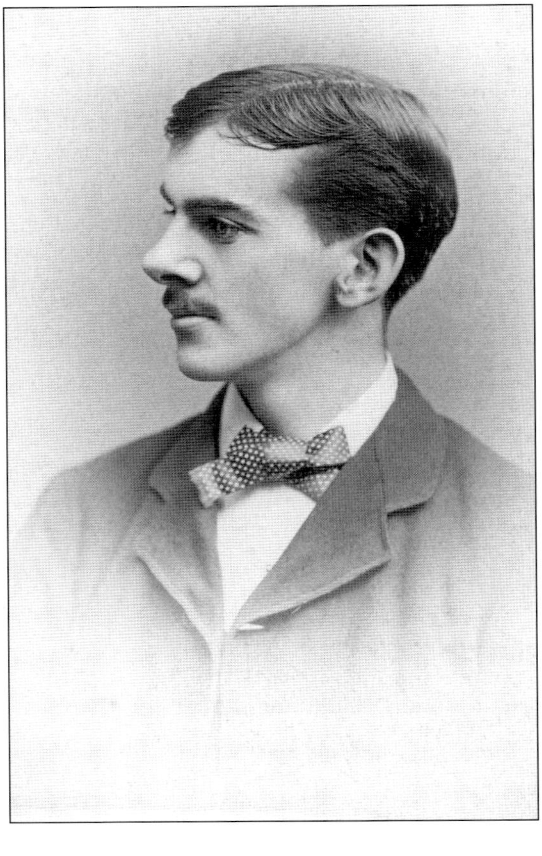

Herbert Collins Parsons was born in Northfield, Massachusetts, in 1862 and by 1889 was an editor at the *Greenfield Gazette and Courier*. He served in the Massachusetts House of Representatives from 1896 to 1898 and in the Massachusetts Senate in 1899. In 1900, he became founder of the *Greenfield Recorder*, succeeded by John Haigis in 1912 when Parsons left Greenfield to become an editorial writer for the *Christian Science Monitor* in Boston. Parsons played a large role in supporting FCPH, particularly in helping to recruit physicians to Greenfield via his many connections in Boston. (NHS.)

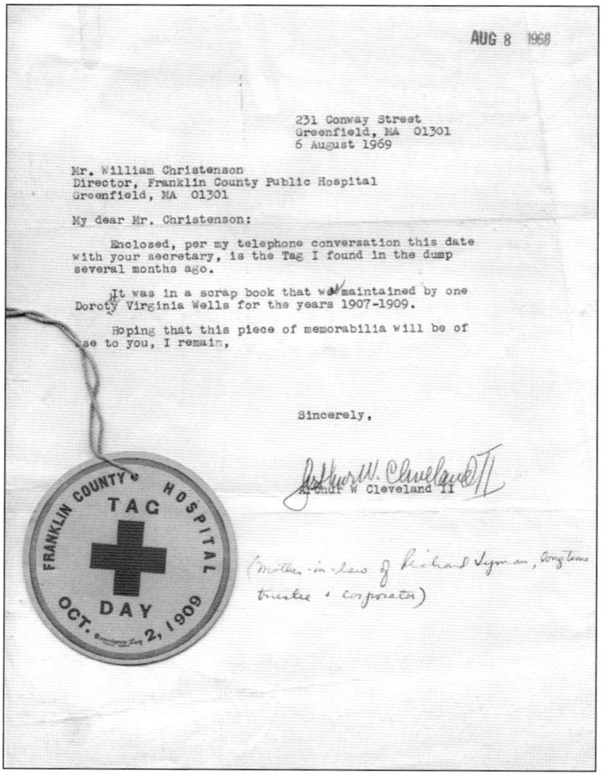

AUG 8 1969

231 Conway Street
Greenfield, MA 01301
6 August 1969

Mr. William Christenson
Director, Franklin County Public Hospital
Greenfield, MA 01301

My dear Mr. Christenson:

Enclosed, per my telephone conversation this date with your secretary, is the Tag I found in the dump several months ago.

It was in a scrap book that was maintained by one Dorothy Virginia Wells for the years 1907-1909.

Hoping that this piece of memorabilia will be of use to you, I remain,

Sincerely,

Arthur W Cleveland II

(mother-in-law of Richard Lyman, longtime trustee + corporator)

Tag Days were popular fundraising traditions for many hospitals in the early 1900s. This tag was found in a scrapbook maintained by Dorothy Virginia Wells of Greenfield, who was the mother-in-law of Richard Lyman, a longtime trustee of FCPH. Tags were worn by hospital supporters to clearly identify them as they took to the streets one day each year to collect money for the hospital. This tag is dated October 2, 1909. It was made by the Dennison Manufacturing Company of Framingham, Massachusetts.

The Converse House had originally been a private home owned by James Converse, a Pennsylvania business executive who chose Greenfield for his retirement. The building functioned as a hospital from 1898 to 1910. After the hospital moved to High Street, this property became an inn and a boarding house, and was demolished in 1950.

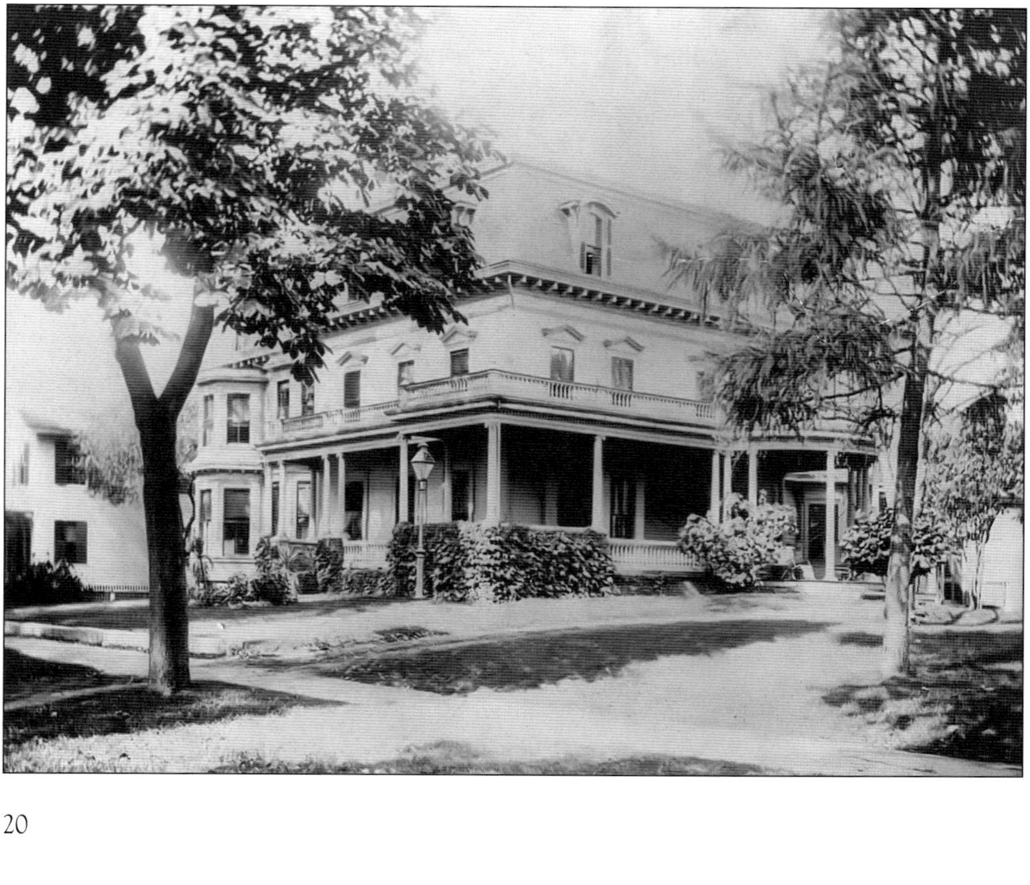

Two

MOVING TO HIGH STREET

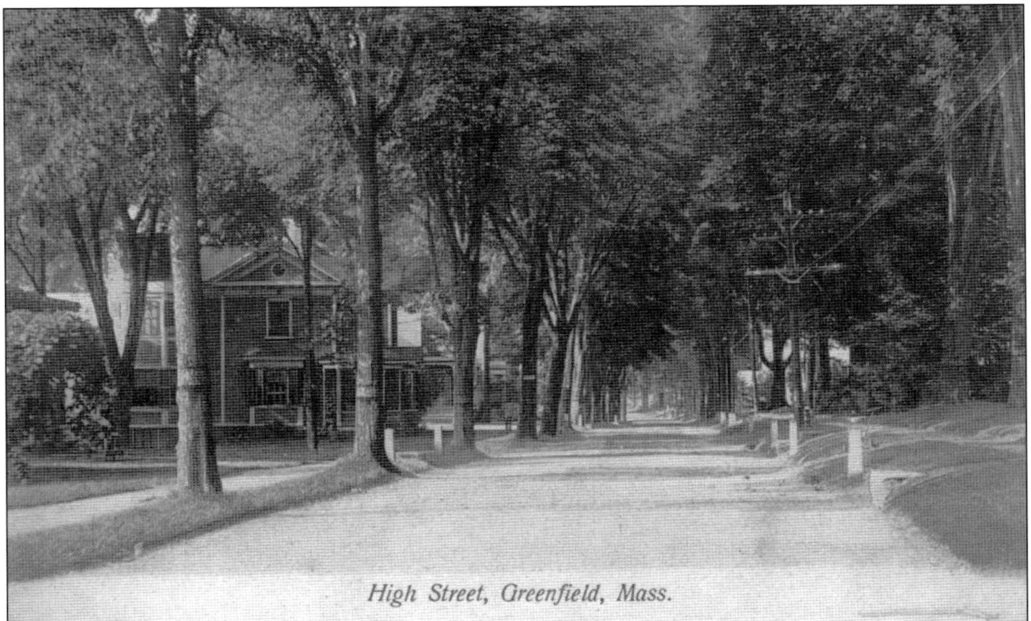

This postcard view shows High Street in Greenfield around 1903. The pastoral image illustrates the residential nature of High Street when land was purchased for the new hospital in 1904. High Street in Greenfield was originally Massachusetts Route 2, the main east-west motor route from Boston to Albany. Today, this road is designated Massachusetts Route 2A, having been bypassed with a modern highway. In 1906, Drs. H.G. Stetson, F.A. Pond, and J.D. Kiley were named to the building committee and charged with raising $50,000 for construction of a new hospital. The Honorable Levi J. Gunn kicked off the campaign with a gift of $10,000. The hospital's property was augmented by the gift of the lot at the corner of High and Sanderson Streets (estimated value of $1,000) by Mrs. John Sheldon and Mrs. George Sheldon. (GOC.)

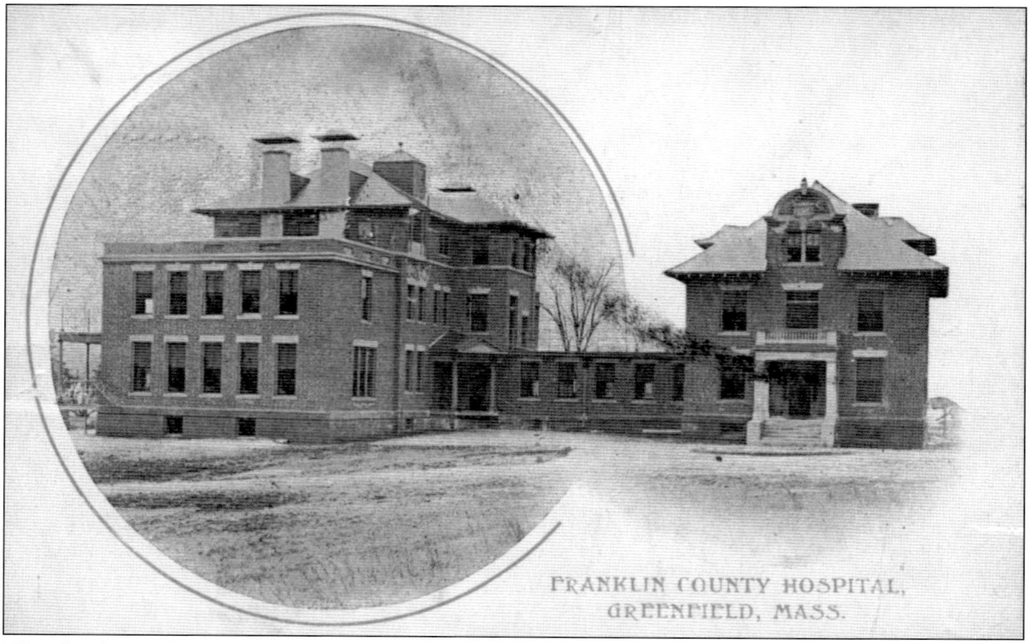

The fundraising committee, chaired by Charles Stoddard and including Dr. G.P. Twitchell, Judge F.N. Thompson, Frank P. Forbes, and Walter S. Carson, successfully raised enough money to construct the new facilities, which were opened in 1910. Two buildings were constructed: the Administration Building and a larger building, known as the South Building, with both private patient rooms and wards. This postcard view of the Franklin County Public Hospital was taken in 1911. Note the open walkway on the roof of the connector. The building to the right is the Administration Building. In 1909, the sale of the Converse House on Main Street had added $9,000 to the hospital's funds. (GOC.)

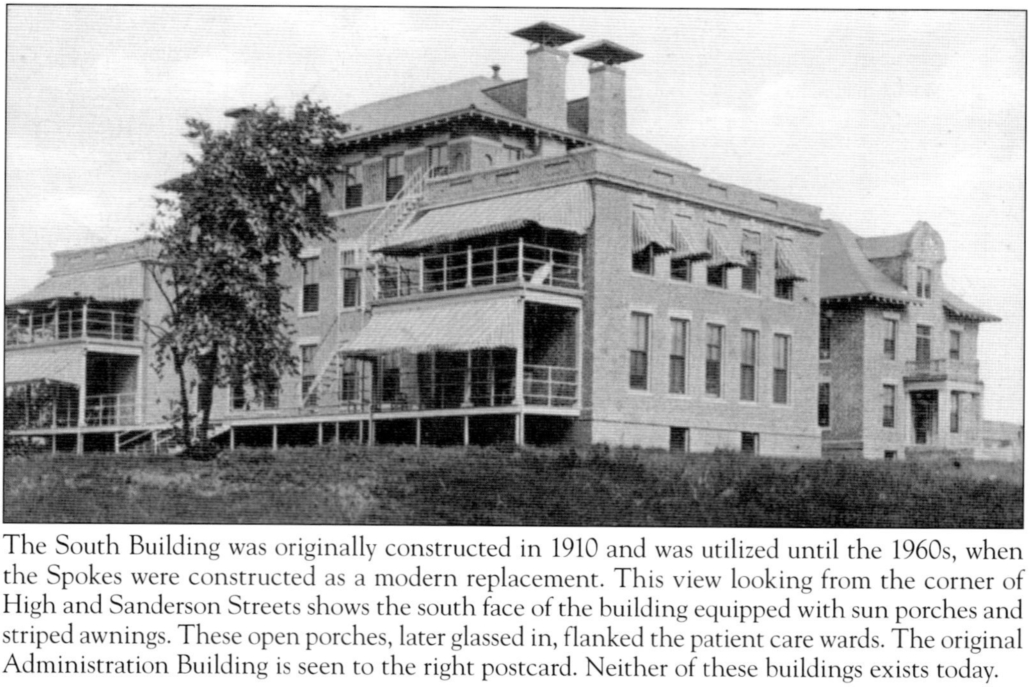

The South Building was originally constructed in 1910 and was utilized until the 1960s, when the Spokes were constructed as a modern replacement. This view looking from the corner of High and Sanderson Streets shows the south face of the building equipped with sun porches and striped awnings. These open porches, later glassed in, flanked the patient care wards. The original Administration Building is seen to the right postcard. Neither of these buildings exists today.

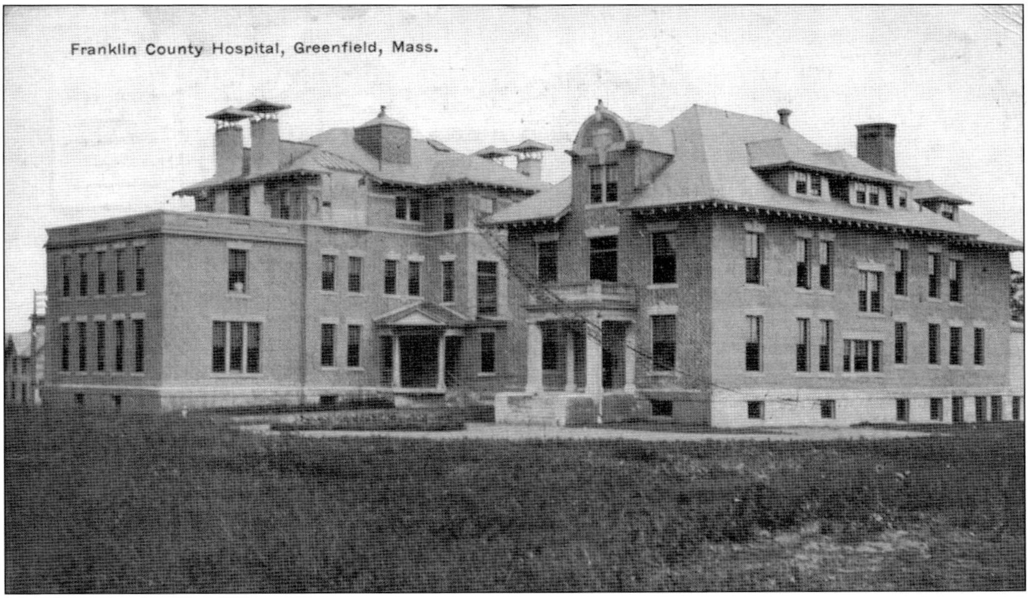
Franklin County Hospital, Greenfield, Mass.

This undated postcard was likely taken as construction was completed. Awnings seen in a similar 1911 postcard view have not yet been added. In this picture, taken from the corner of High Street and Beacon Street, the South Building is on the left, and the third floor features large north-facing windows to admit light for the operating room. This structure was torn down in the mid-1960s after construction of the Spokes. The Administration Building, to the right, was torn down to accommodate the new Central Building, added in 1952. The two buildings were connected by an enclosed walkway on the first floor and an open walkway on the second. (TLH.)

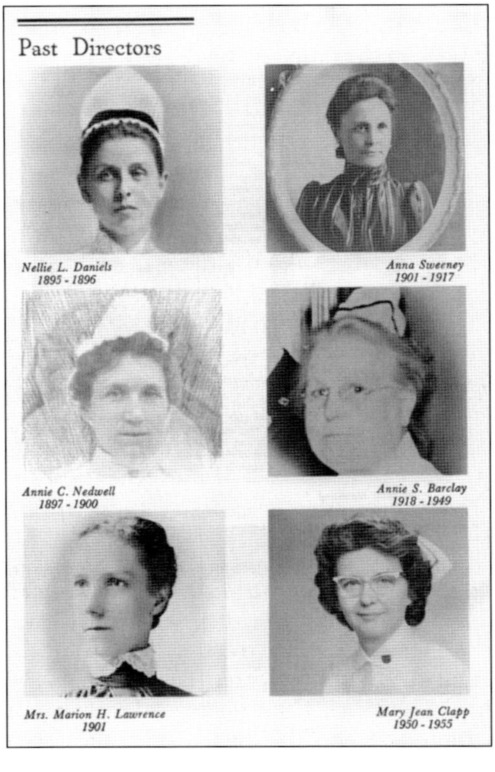
Past Directors
Nellie L. Daniels
1895 - 1896
Anna Sweeney
1901 - 1917
Annie C. Nedwell
1897 - 1900
Annie S. Barclay
1918 - 1949
Mrs. Marion H. Lawrence
1901
Mary Jean Clapp
1950 - 1955

Six nurses held the title of director of nursing between 1895 and 1955: Nellie L. Daniels, Annie Nedwell, Marion Lawrence, Anna Sweeney, Annie Barclay, and Mary Jean Clapp. Nellie Daniels was hired as superintendent of the hospital when it opened on September 9, 1895. Anna Moritz was the first student nurse in training. Around the beginning of the 20th century, most hospitals employed only a handful of senior nurses, with most patient care provided by student nurses whose education was primarily hands-on under experienced supervision.

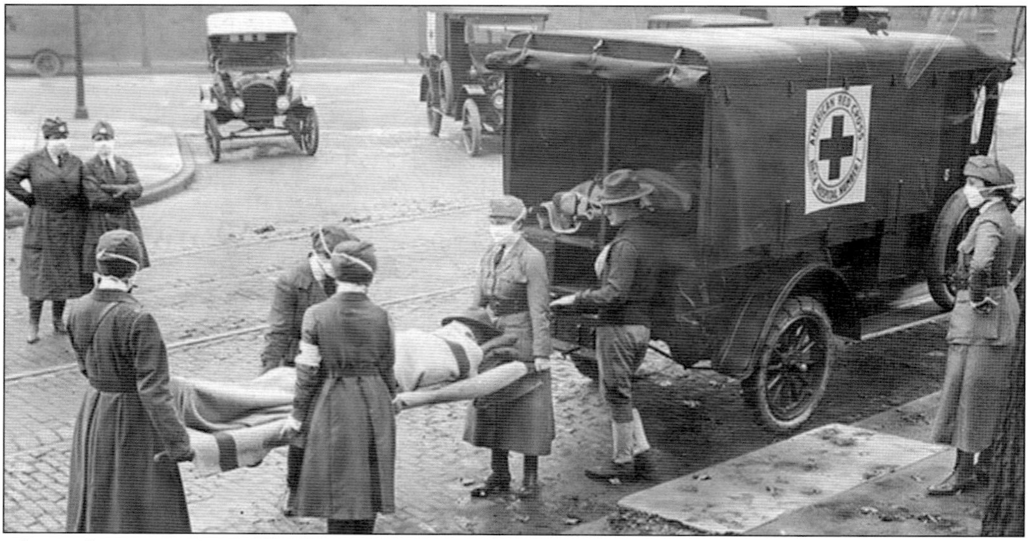

The influenza outbreak of 1918–1919 was particularly devastating in Franklin County, as well as in Massachusetts (45,000 died). In the United States, 675,000 died. Worldwide, the "Spanish Flu" took more victims than were claimed by World War I. Western Massachusetts began seeing cases in October 1918, presumably spread by sailors returning through the port of Boston. The Greenfield Board of Health ordered theaters, schools, churches, libraries, and clubs closed and forbade assemblages of people. Physicians and nurses fell ill, complicating an existing shortage due to the World War. Between September 26 and October 4, 1918, there were 340 cases in Greenfield, with 16 deaths, including two nurses. Up to 10 patients were admitted to FCPH each day, with six deaths on one day. Within 36 hours of a board directive, the "south piazza" was roofed over so that more patients could be accommodated. During the height of the epidemic, 135 patients were admitted with 46 deaths, an astounding 34 percent mortality rate. This photograph appeared in a historical review published by the *Greenfield Recorder* on December 18, 2001. (GR.)

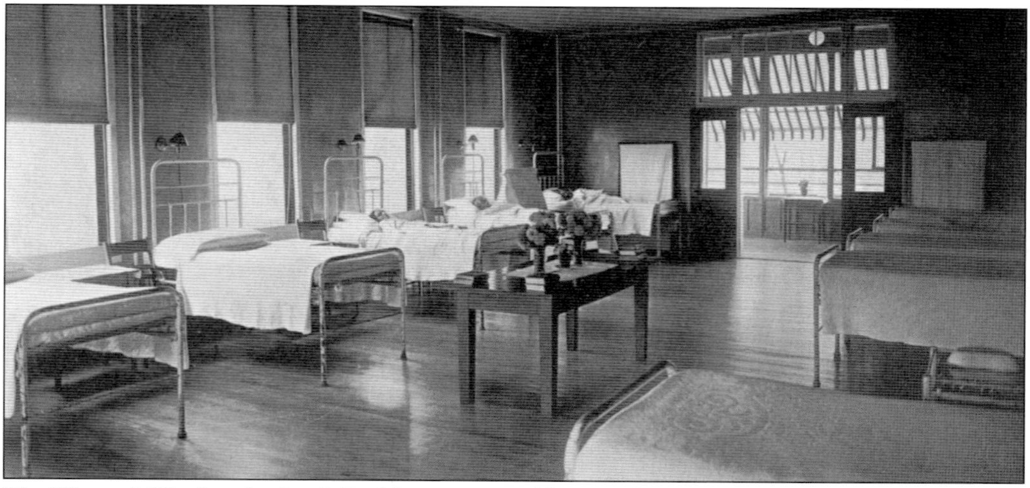

The Women's Ward in the South Building is pictured here. A dozen patients could be accommodated with beds flanking five windows on each side. The sun porch and awning are visible, along with portable screens that could be wheeled into place between beds when privacy was warranted. FCPH's capacity was overwhelmed by the influenza epidemic, and in direct response, the town of Greenfield opened the region's first isolation hospital in 1922, located in the Sanderson Building, separate from FCPH but on the grounds and under the hospital's direct supervision.

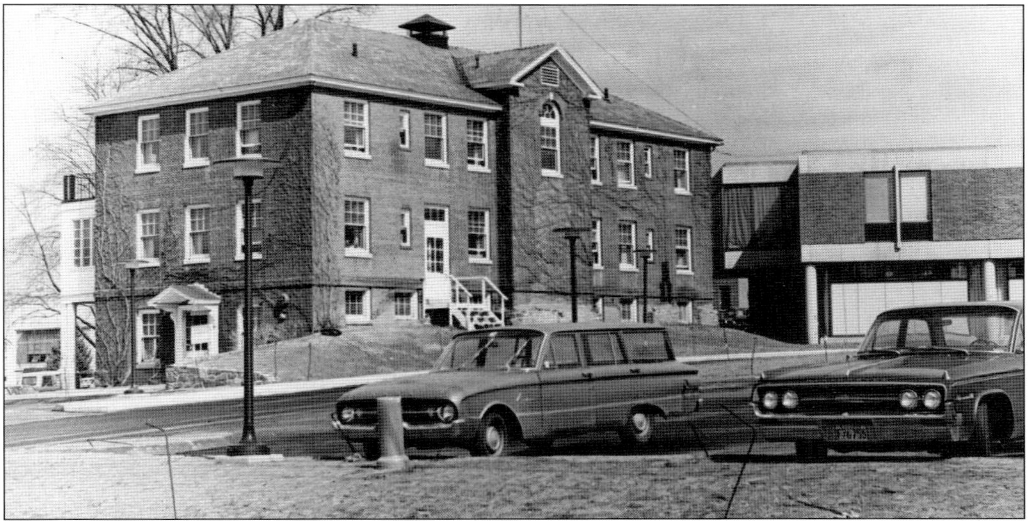

Surprisingly few photographs exist of the isolation hospital, also known as the Sanderson Building. The structure was completed in 1922, operated by the town as an isolation hospital, and turned over by the town of Greenfield to FCPH in 1955, when it became an alcohol rehabilitation unit. In this view from the late 1960s, the former isolation hospital seems to nearly touch the recently completed Spoke IV. The original facade was extensively modified with removal of a central entrance and conversion of a window to provide emergency egress.

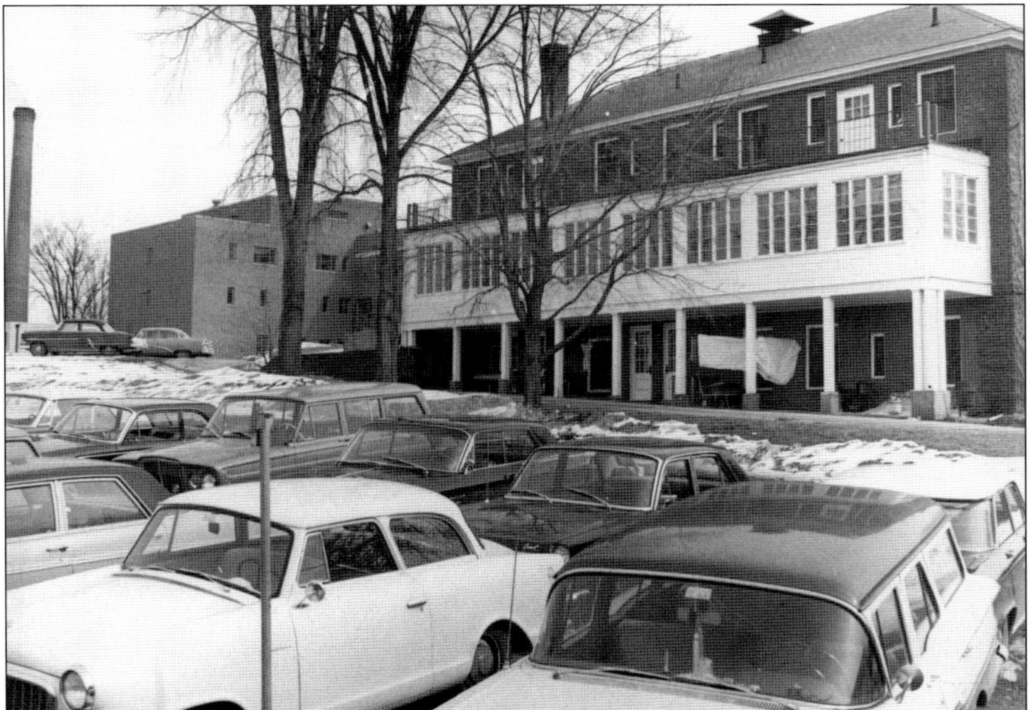

The west (back) face of the Sanderson Building featured an enclosed porch on the first floor and an open porch above. Linens appear to be airing outside the ground level. The cars in the employees' parking lot date this picture to the early 1960s. This building was torn down in 2005 to enlarge the Sanderson Street parking lot.

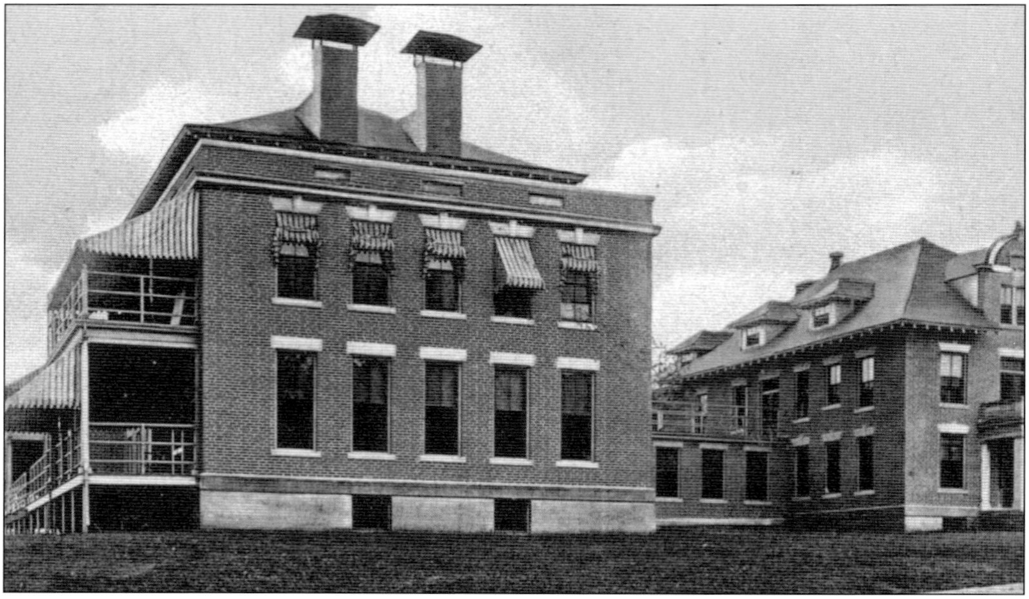

In this postcard view of the hospital from High Street, striped awnings have been added. The porches were enclosed to increase capacity after the 1918 influenza epidemic. (TLH.)

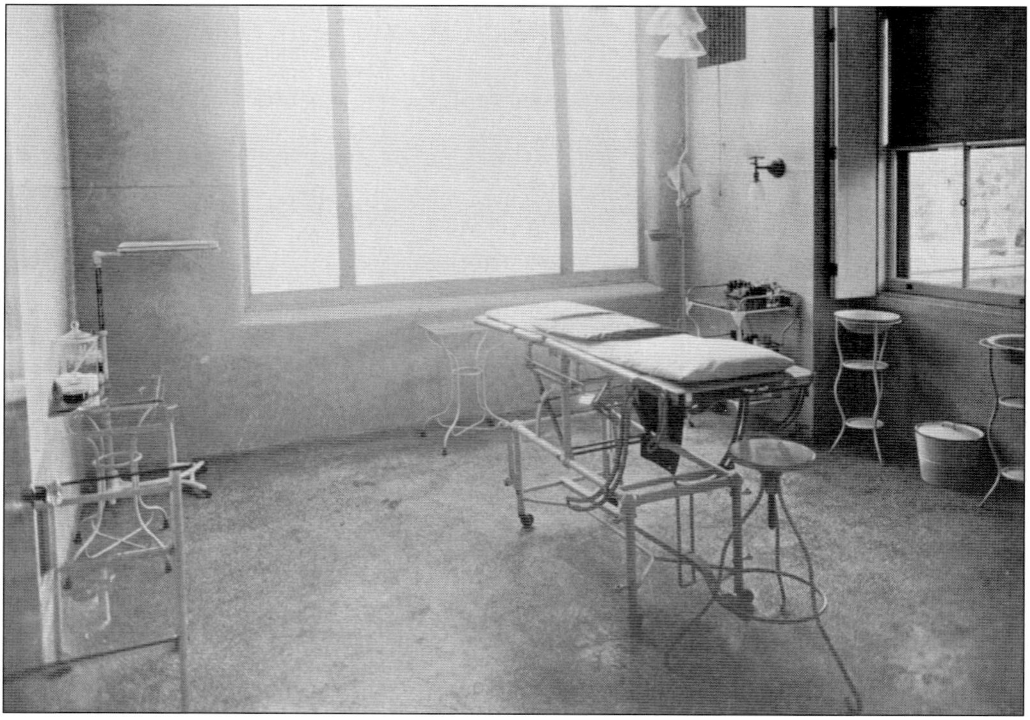

This 1922 photograph was taken in the South Building, prior to the construction of new operating rooms in the 1927 North Building. Some equipment, such as the Mayo instrument stand (to the left of the window), would be familiar today. The basin stands (under the right window) and two overhead pendant lamps appear rather primitive. In the days before modern parabolic lighting fixtures, operating rooms were usually built with large, north-facing windows that took advantage of ambient light without the heat and sharp shadows that would accompany south-facing windows.

Annie S. Barclay, RN, was born in Boston, graduated from Boston City Hospital School of Nursing, and served with the Red Cross in England for 14 months during World War I. She was appointed superintendent of nurses at FCPH in 1916, serving in that position until her retirement in 1949. She was also named hospital superintendent in 1918, succeeding Anna Sweeney, who had held that position from 1901 to 1917. It was early in her tenure that the challenging influenza epidemic of 1918 occurred. Barclay was the hospital supervisor from 1918 to 1946.

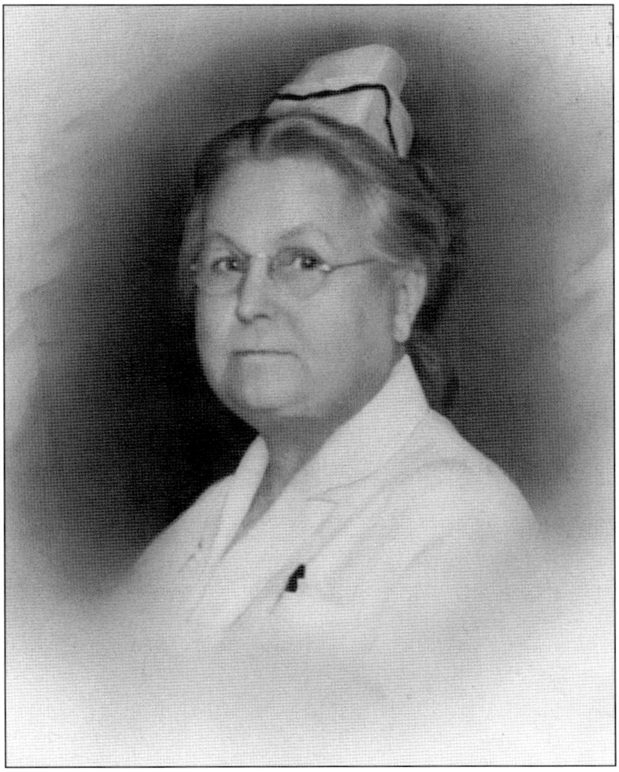

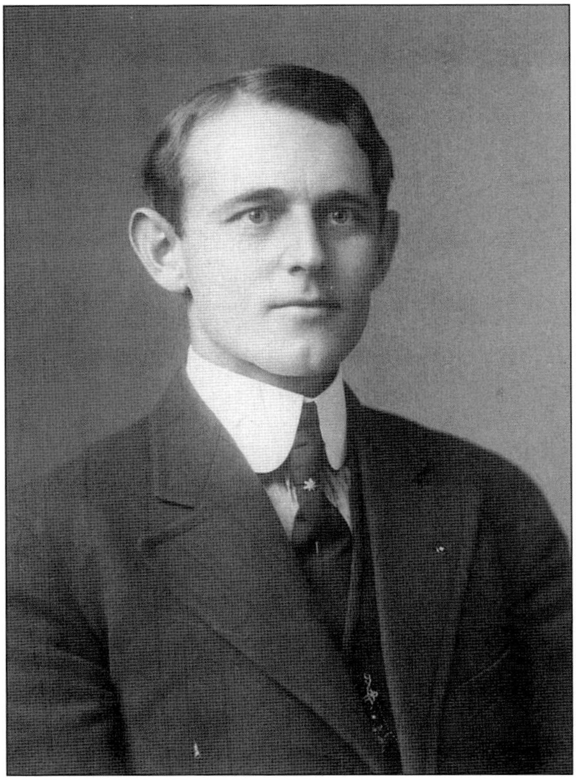

John W. Haigis (1881–1960) was the editor and publisher of the *Greenfield Recorder* and founded the radio station WHAI in Greenfield. His political career included town officer in Montague and election to the Massachusetts House of Representatives and then the Senate. He was also a trustee of the University of Massachusetts. In 1925, Haigis became the chairman of the $300,000 fundraising drive to support construction of the North Building at FCPH and a new dormitory for the nursing school. (GHS.)

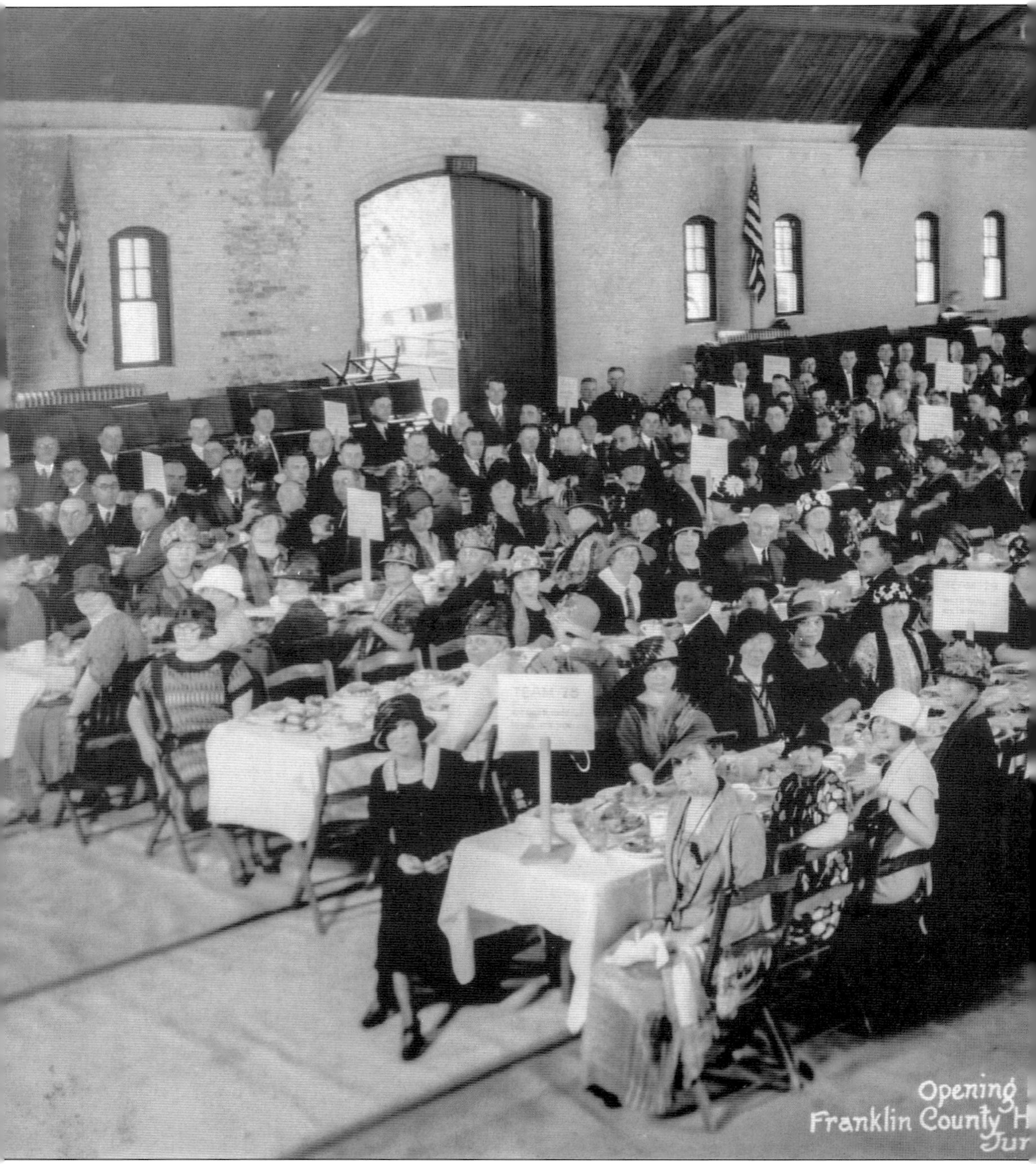

The influenza epidemic of 1918 stretched the hospital's resources nearly to the breaking point. In 1922, a separate Infectious Disease Building was opened adjacent to the hospital, but space remained tight. A fundraising campaign was launched in 1925 to build a new North Building intended to balance the South Building on the opposite side of the central Administration

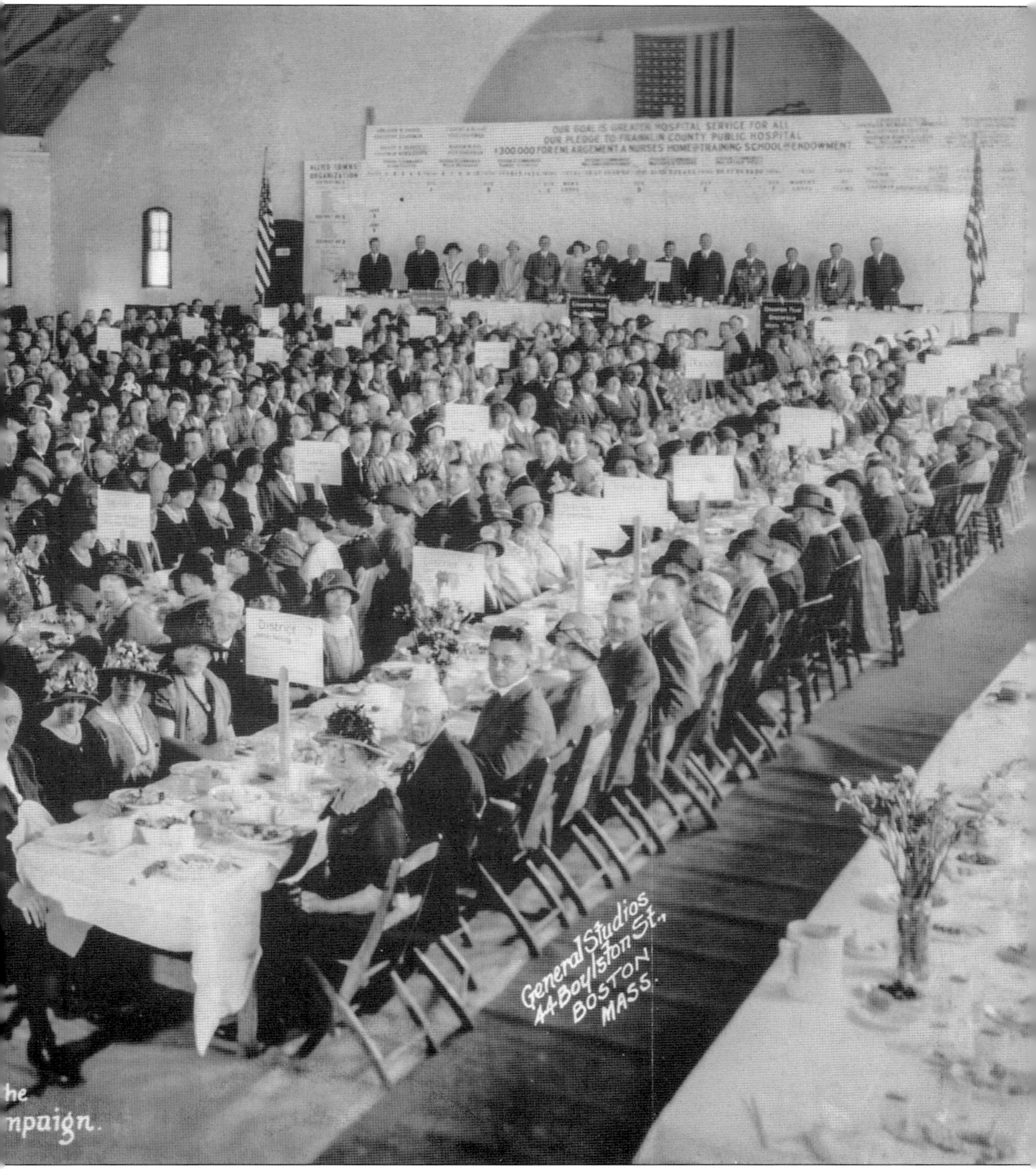
OUR GOAL IS GREATER HOSPITAL SERVICE FOR ALL
OUR PLEDGE TO FRANKLIN COUNTY PUBLIC HOSPITAL
General Studios
44 Boylston St.
BOSTON
MASS.

Building. This photograph shows the opening dinner of the Franklin County Public Hospital Campaign on June 1, 1925. Over 400 people attended this event; they are pictured here divided into fundraising teams.

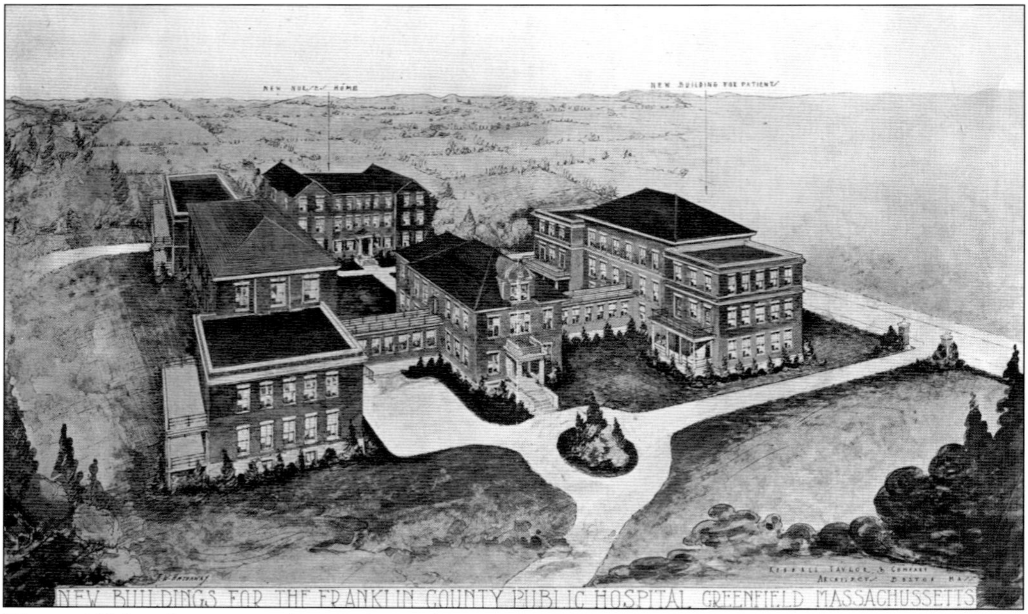

This c. 1925 architect's rendering shows the proposed new North Building and new Nurses Home. To the left is the existing South Building, built in 1910 and connected by an enclosed corridor to the central Administrative Building. Beacon Street is visible behind the proposed new North Building, which, along with the new residence for the nursing school, was completed in 1927.

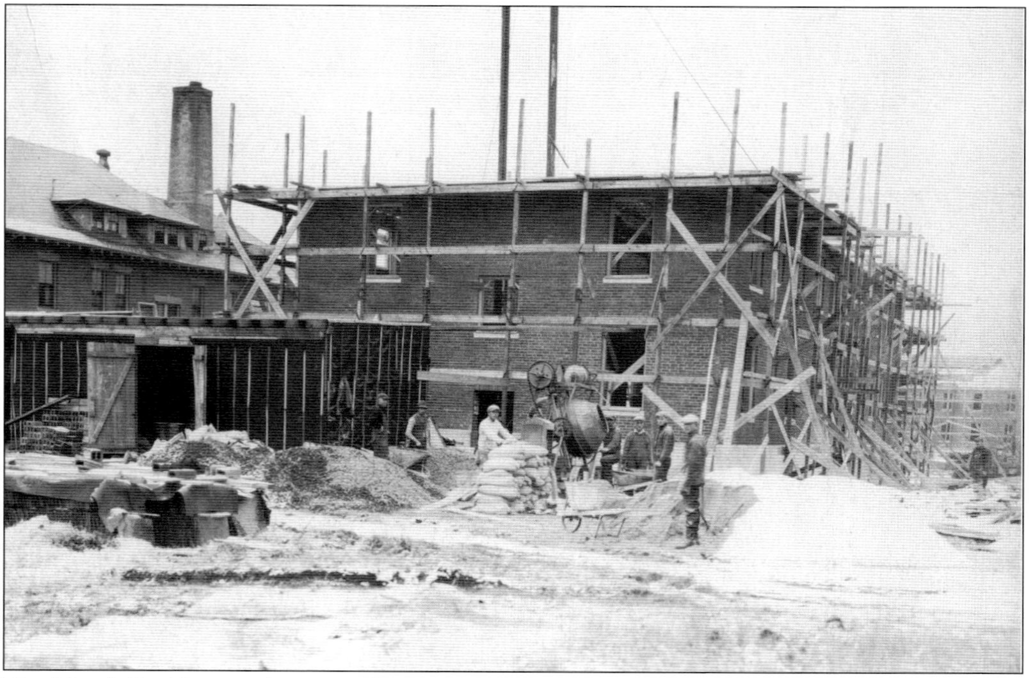

The North Building is shown under construction in 1926. This project, made possible by the 1925 fundraising drive, increased the inpatient capacity from 50 to 100 and allowed the addition of a clinical laboratory and better facilities for the Radiology Department. This new building also accommodated the 1928 collaboration between FCPH and the Farren Memorial Hospital to establish a cancer clinic, a progressive development for its time.

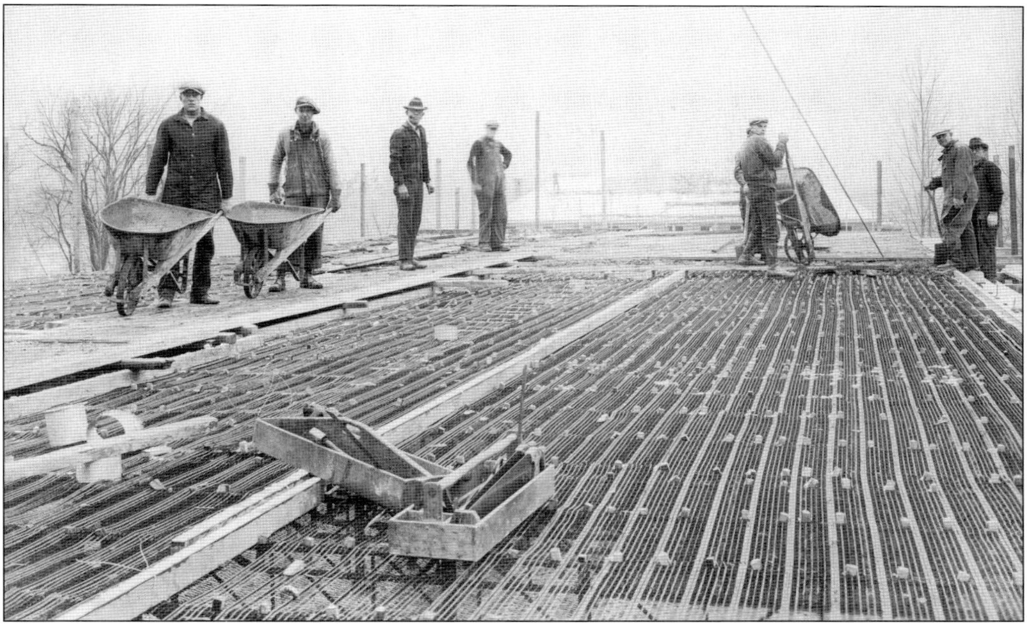

Workmen pour the concrete that will become the third floor of the new North Building. While this building is no longer used for inpatient care, it remains today and is occupied by administrative offices on the first and second floor and support areas for the obstetrics program on the third floor.

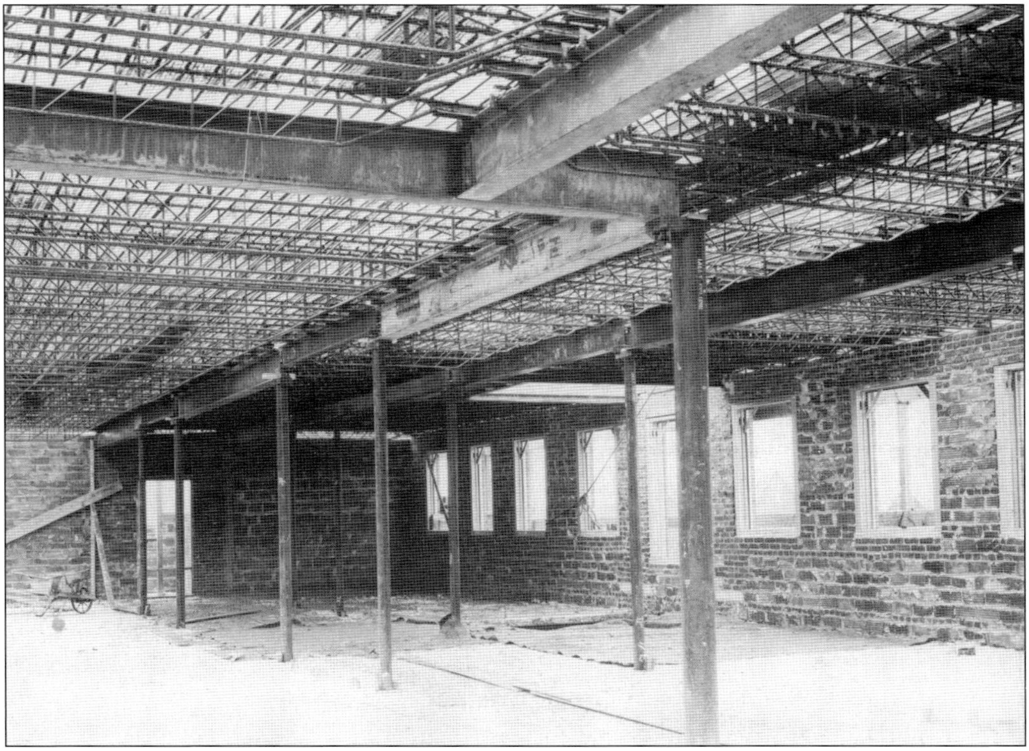

This image is from the interior of the second floor of the North Building facing Beacon Street as the building was being constructed in 1926. The sturdily constructed building remains today, with many of the rooms that were used for patients now repurposed as offices and classrooms.

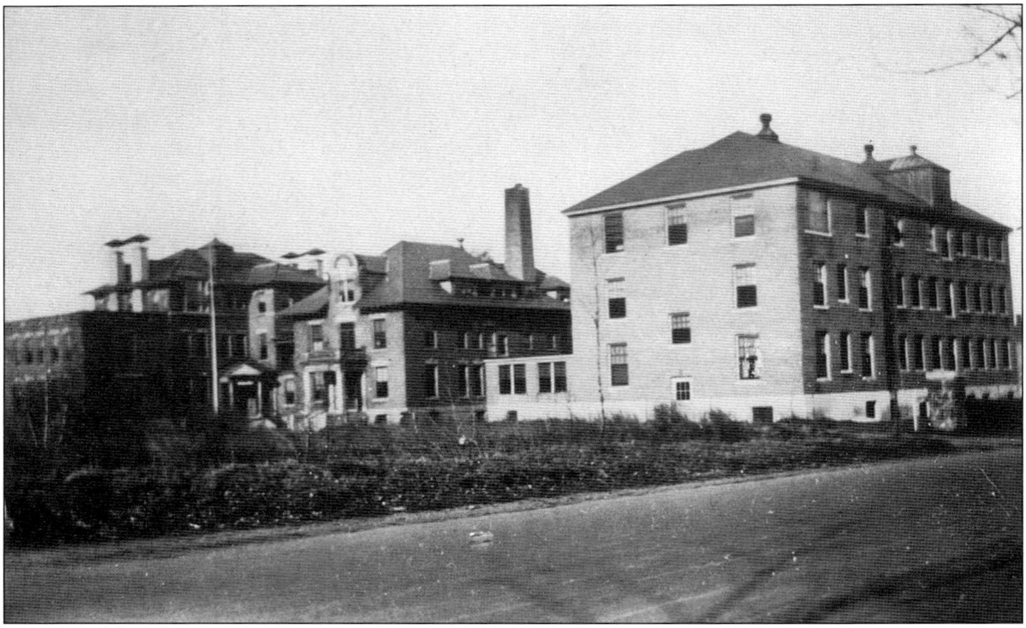

The North Building, completed in 1927, is shown around 1948. At that time, it was connected to the original Administration Building via an enclosed walkway. The walkway and the Administration Building were replaced with the 1952 construction of what is now called the Central Building.

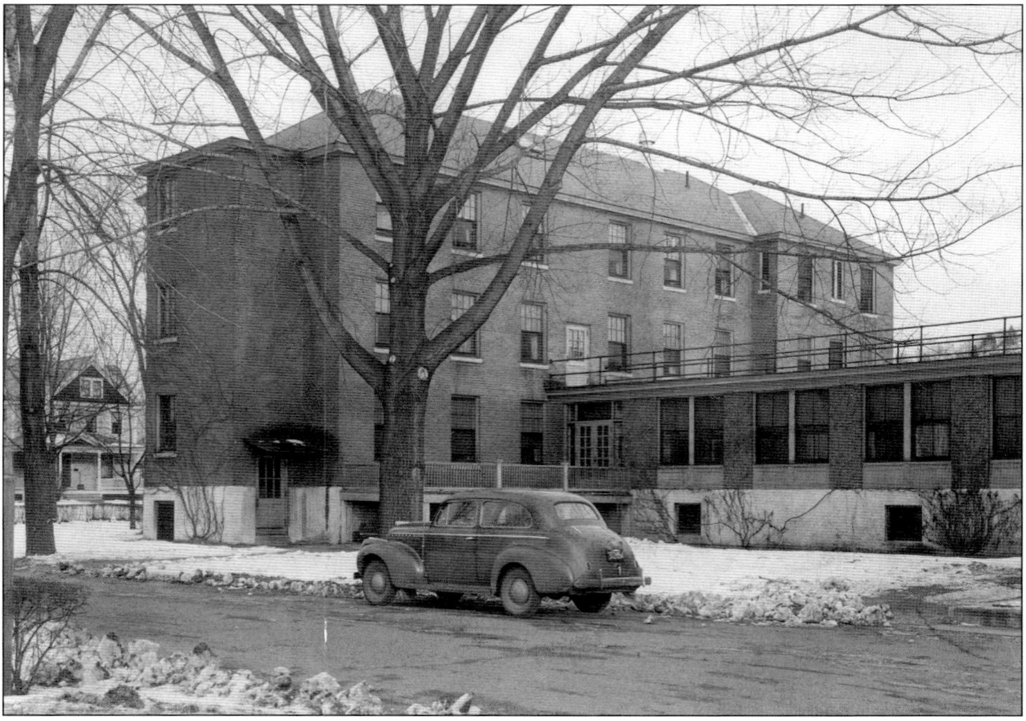

This photograph of the south and west sides of the North Building, also called the North Wing, was taken in March 1948. Also visible is the house on Beacon Street that was torn down in later years for the creation of the Beacon Street parking lot. Much of the south side of this building was connected to the new Central Building in 1952.

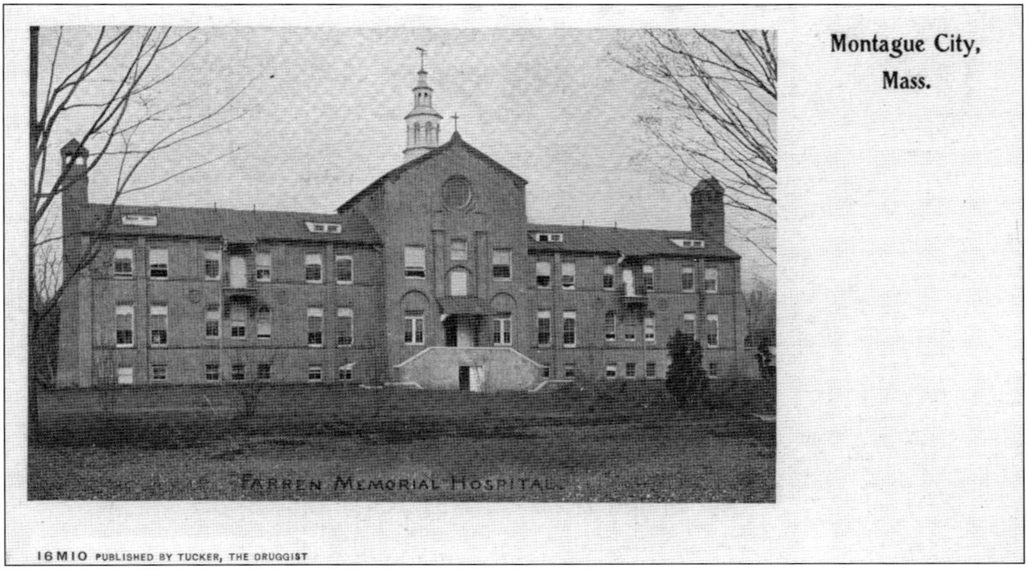

Additional clinical facilities in the North Building facilitated collaboration between FCPH and the Farren Memorial Hospital for cancer care. Beginning in 1928, the two hospitals held joint cancer detection clinics. The Farren was located in Montague City, across the Connecticut River from Greenfield. Montague citizen Barney Farren spearheaded the creation of a community hospital in 1900 that was later named in his honor. Farren Memorial Hospital was an independent entity until 1984, when it was acquired by Providence Systems, later Sisters of Providence Health Systems. In 1988, the hospital was converted into a long-term care facility, and it still stands today. (PVMA.)

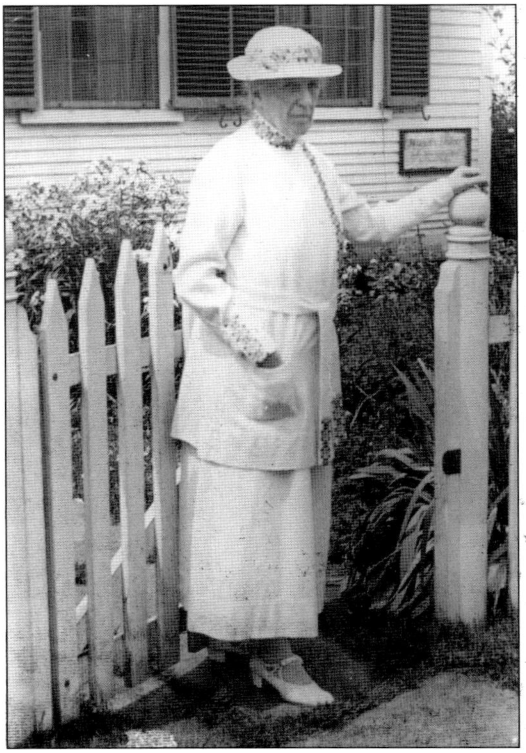

Dr. Mary Phylinda Dole, thought to be the first female physician at FCPH, was born in Shelburne, Massachusetts, in 1862. After attending Sanderson Academy and Mount Holyoke College, she graduated in 1888 from the Women's Medical College of Baltimore. Before moving to Greenfield in 1891, she practiced in Shelburne Falls and at the New England Hospital for Women and Children in Boston. Her private practice was located in the Hovey House, now the Greenfield Public Library. Following her retirement in 1906, she had a second career as a weaver at the Indian House Memorial in Deerfield. She died at age 84 in 1947 and is buried at the East Shelburne Cemetery. (PVMA.)

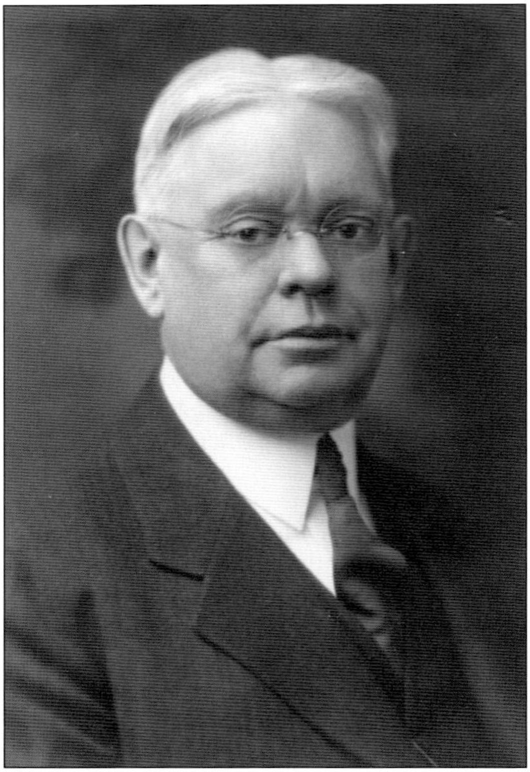

Dr. Halbert G. Stetson (1868–1943) had a long and productive history with FCPH, including service as president of the board of trustees from 1917 to 1920 and 1937 to 1943. Stetson attended the College of Physicians and Surgeons in Baltimore, Maryland, receiving his medical degree in April 1895. He returned to Greenfield, where his practice soon concentrated on surgery. He was a member of the Springfield Academy of Medicine, the New England Surgical Society, and the Greenfield Board of Health. He was chairman of the school board, president of the chamber of commerce, president of the Massachusetts Medical Society in 1931, and a member of the American Hospital Association and the Greenfield Doctor's Club. Stetson was one of the inspiring and leading spirits of the hospital for some 40 years. He was married on June 30, 1897, to Francis A. Gildart of Salisbury, New Brunswick. After becoming a widower in 1920, he then married Annabelle Mackenzie of Greenfield. He is buried at the Green River Cemetery in Greenfield.

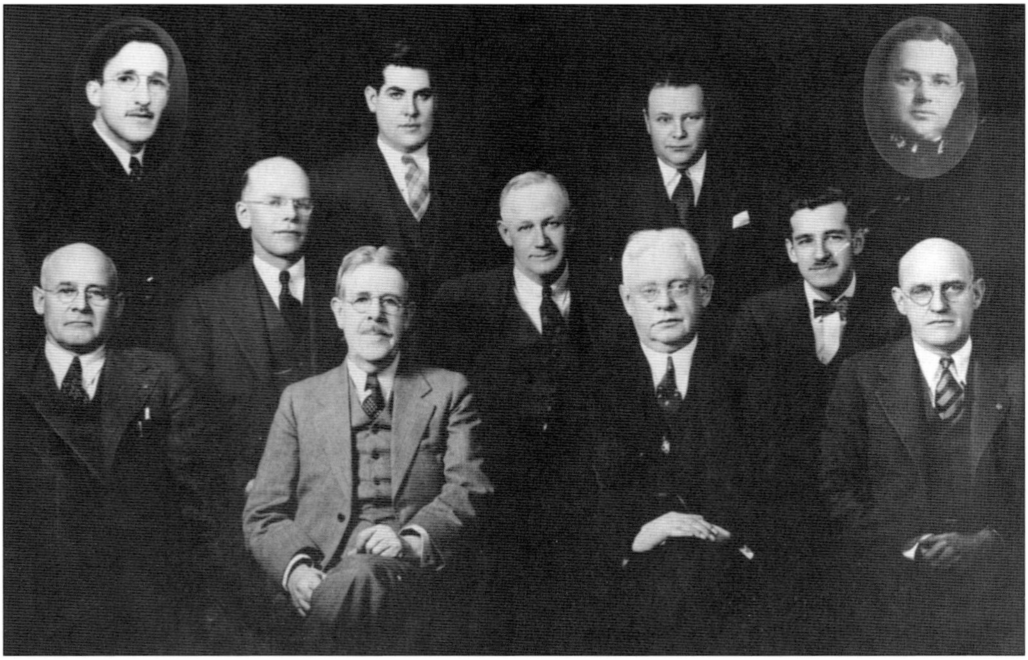

FCPH's medical staff is pictured in the early 1930s. The physician in the upper left inset is Chauncey V. Perry, who died in 1936. Seated in the first row are Dr. R.S. Russell of Deerfield (left center) and Dr. Halbert G. Stetson (right center). In 1938; Dr. Stetson was elected president of the hospital; shortly after this time, FCPH became one of the first institutions to accept insurance payments.

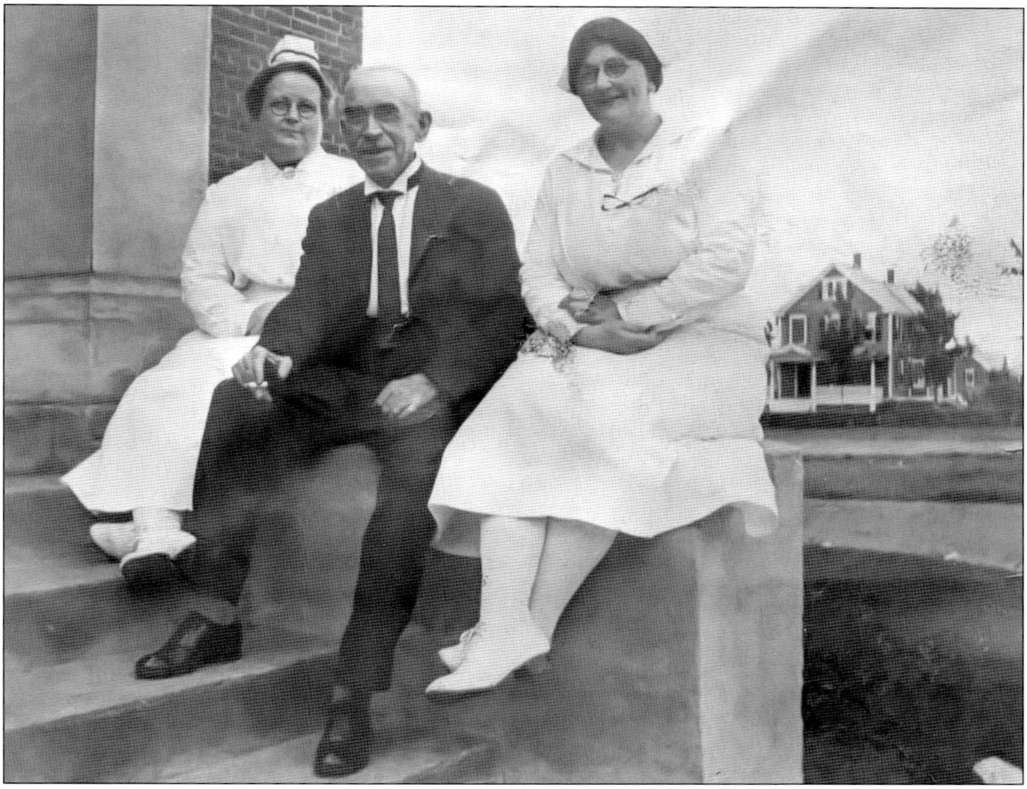

Dr. George P. Twitchell is pictured in 1919 on the steps of FCPH along with two nurses. He specialized in obstetrics and was also a medical examiner in Franklin County during his tenure.

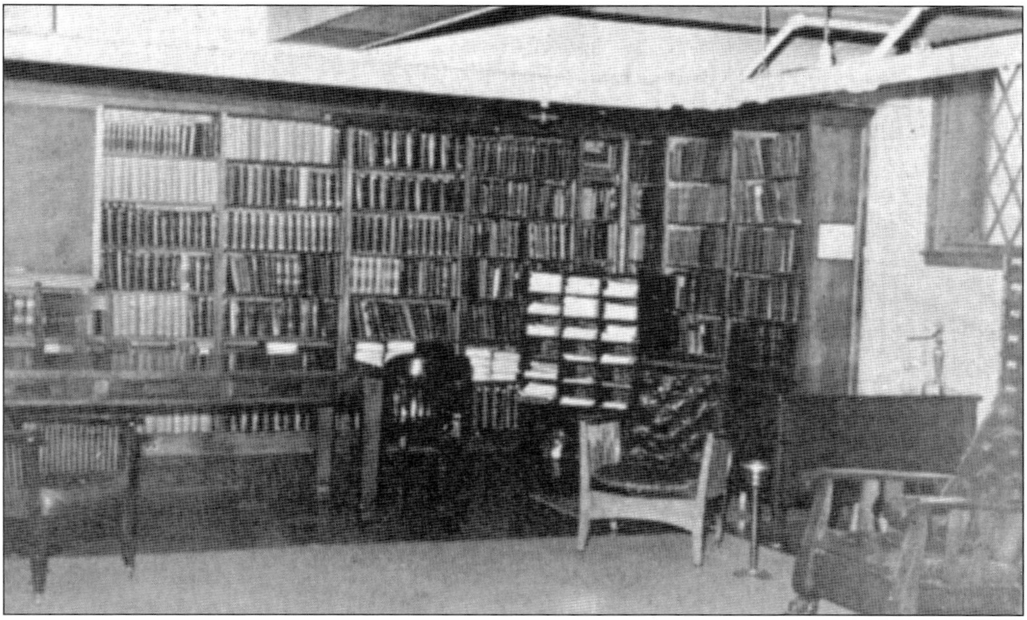

The Twitchell-Canedy Library, a local medical reference center for staff physicians, was gifted to FCPH by Dr. Halbert G. Stetson in December 1938 in memory of his long-standing associates Dr. George P. Twitchell, who passed away in 1930, and Dr. Charles F. Canedy, who passed away in 1925.

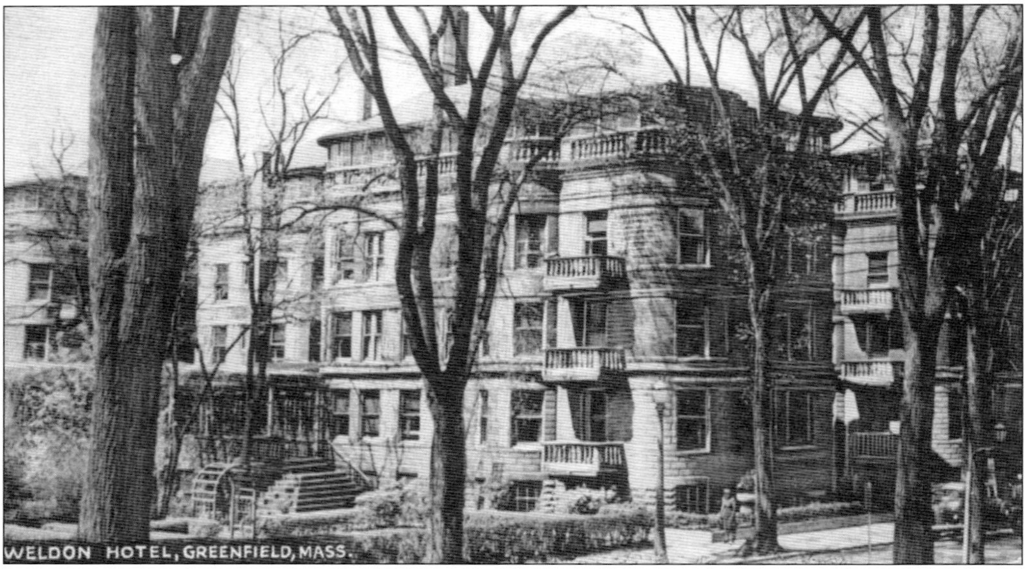

The Weldon Hotel, located near FCPH on High Street, was built in 1905 by F.O. Wells, who was determined to build the most innovative structure in Greenfield. The Weldon was one of the first poured concrete buildings and was the first all-concrete hotel in New England. While originally designed for company suites and residential apartments, in 1907, it became a high-end hotel for overnight lodging. During its heyday, it hosted numerous hospital social events. (TLH.)

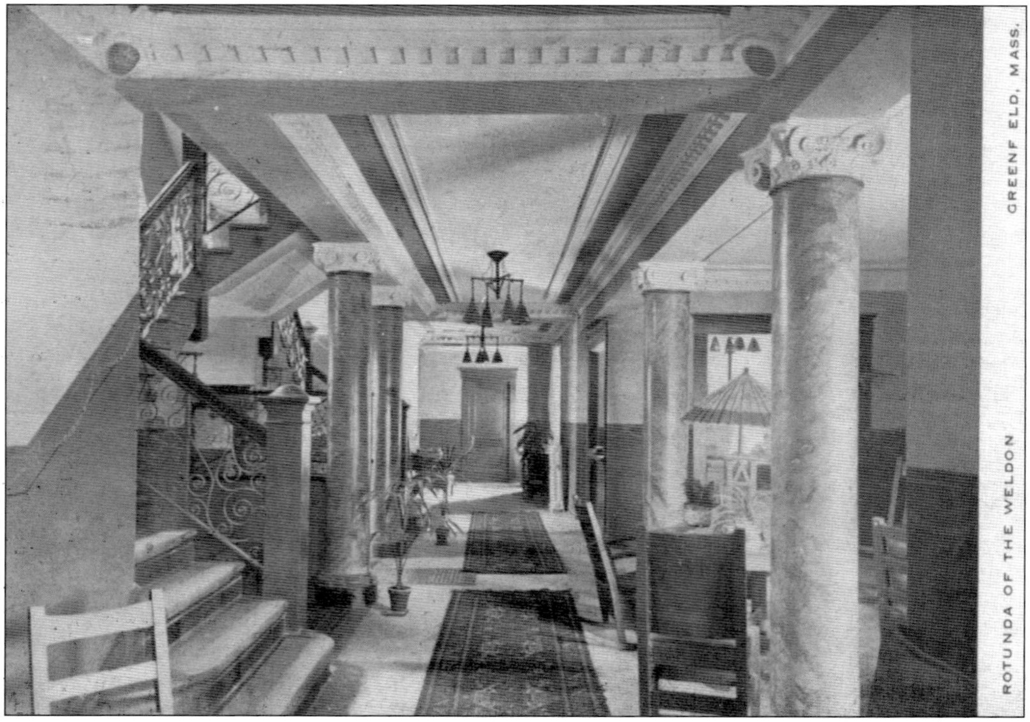

The Weldon Hotel, located on Massachusetts Route 2 (the Mohawk Trail), was a popular tourist destination year round, featuring hiking and skiing in nearby Highland Park. The rotunda of the hotel is pictured in this 1909 postcard. With the opening of the Route 2 bypass, business declined, and the hotel closed in 1977. Today it is a senior living facility. (TLH.)

Dr. Chauncey Valentine Perry (1900–1936) was a surgeon on the FCPH medical staff from 1931 to 1936. He was a 1928 Harvard Medical School graduate who interned at Boston City Hospital. He died in December 1936 at the age of 36 as a result of an accidental overdose of morphine. His body was discovered at the nearby Weldon Hotel.

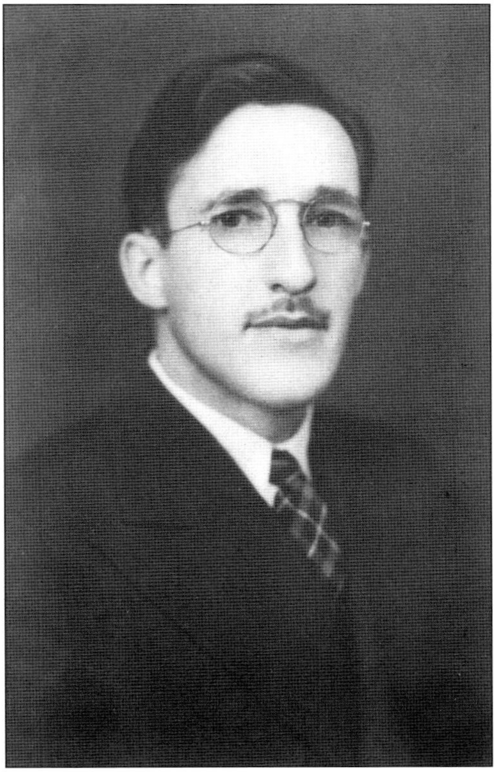

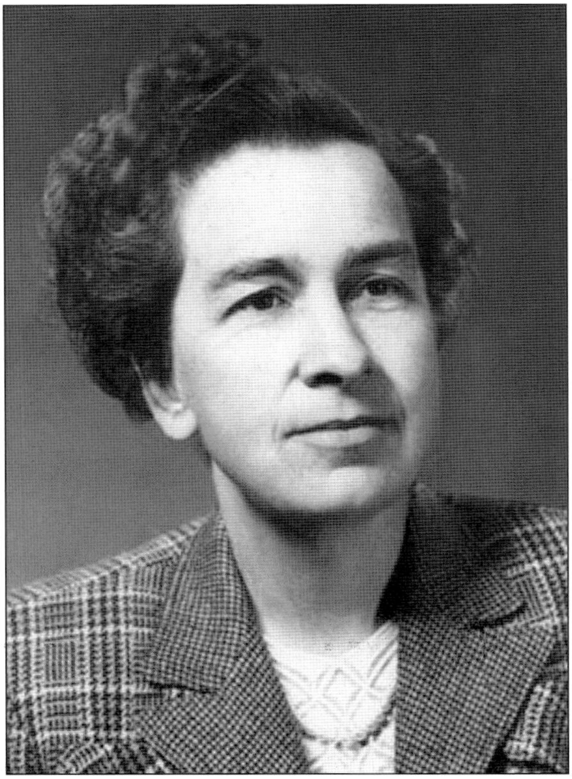

Harriet Louise Hardy (1906–1993) was recruited to Franklin County in 1937 to start a much-needed heart clinic. Dr. Hardy was working at the Northfield Seminary for Girls when the Hurricane of 1938 hit Franklin County. A two-ton chimney fell through the roof of Gould Hall, injuring many of the 100 students who were eating dinner, with two students dying. With the Connecticut River flooded, which blocked access to FCPH, and many of the local physicians out of town for hunting season, Dr. Hardy and her nurse worked feverishly to set bones and sew up lacerations by lantern light. This natural disaster forced her into taking an extended leave due to exhaustion and depression. After leaving the Greenfield area in 1939, she became the first female associate clinical professor of medicine at Harvard in 1958 and founded the national beryllium registry. (Courtesy of the National Library of Medicine.)

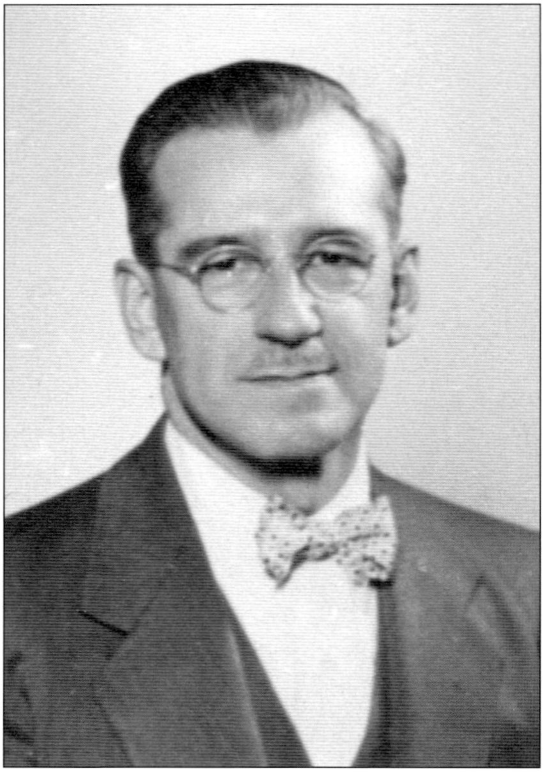

Dr. Lawrence Dame was born in 1901 in Malden, Massachusetts, and died in 1974 while on a trip to Wisconsin, but he is buried in Green River Cemetery in Greenfield. He was president of the Massachusetts Medical Society from 1959 to 1960, one of four FCPH physicians who held this position, in addition to being president of the Franklin District Medical Society. He began his career in Shelburne Falls as a general practitioner but later went on to specialize in ophthalmology.

The South Building is pictured with a late 1940s automobile ignoring the no parking signs in front of the ambulance entrance. The large glass window on the third floor admitted light for an operating room. Note the sign over the doorway that reads "Night Entrance." This was also the entrance that was used for ambulances.

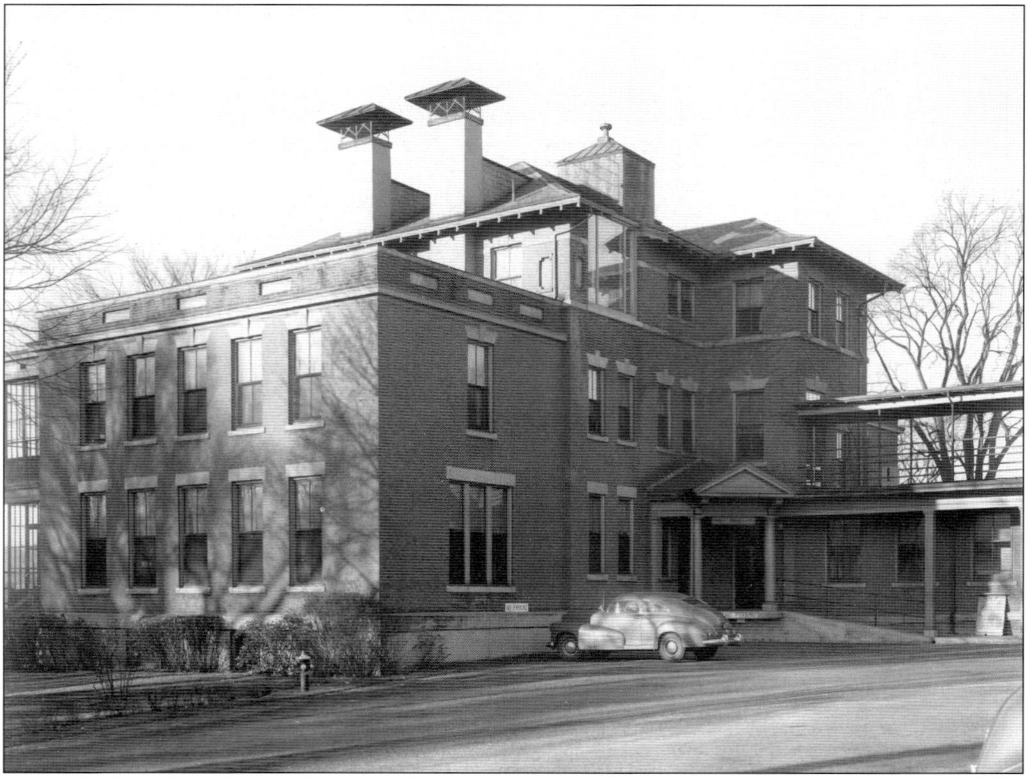

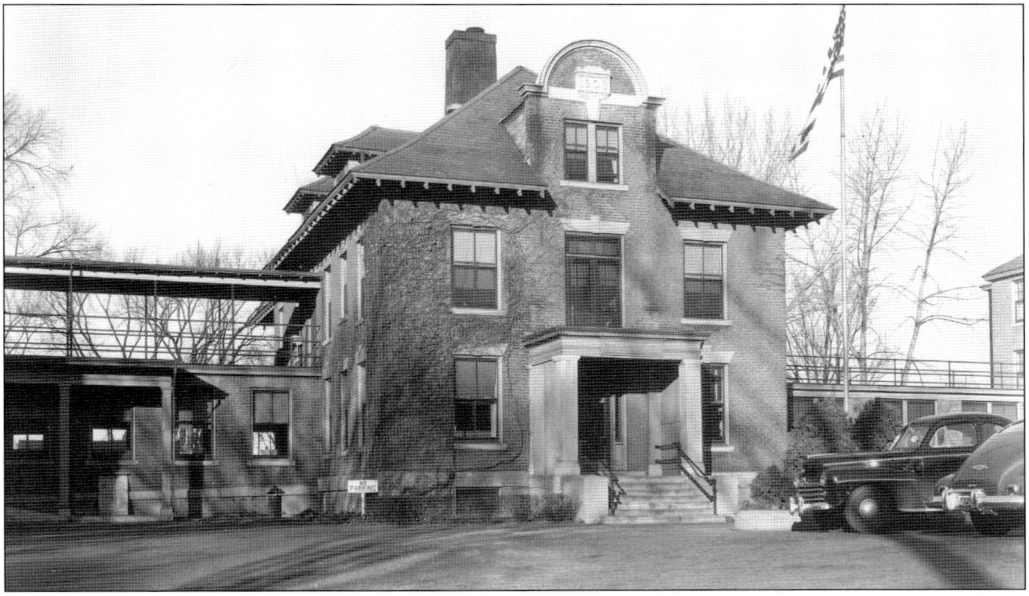

Although the hospital opened its High Street location in 1910, the date over the third floor of the Administration Building's top window reads 1908, the year construction was started. The cars date this photograph to the late 1940s or early 1950s, prior to construction of the new Central Building, which was completed in 1952. The open corridor that led to the second floor of the former South Building can be seen on the left, while the North Building (which still remains today) is visible at far right.

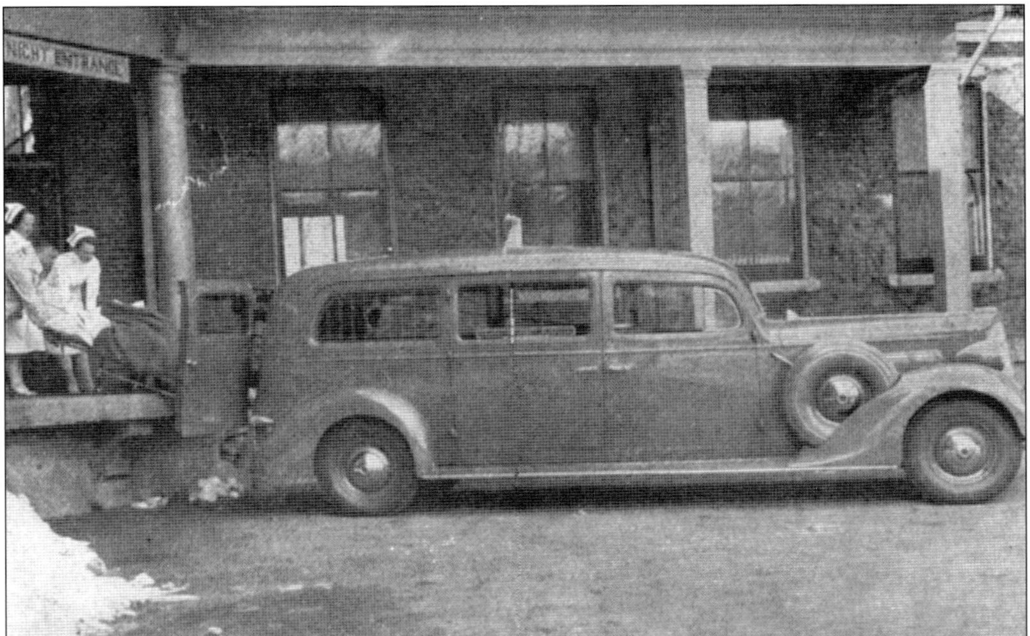

In this 1945 photograph, nurses Miss Ellis and Mrs. Poirier wheel a patient from the ambulance dock to the emergency room, then located on the north side of the South Building, also known as 1 South. The money for this ambulance was given by Alice Judd, a local resident of Greenfield who had ties to the Judd Paper Company in Holyoke. (Courtesy of Doug Lyman.)

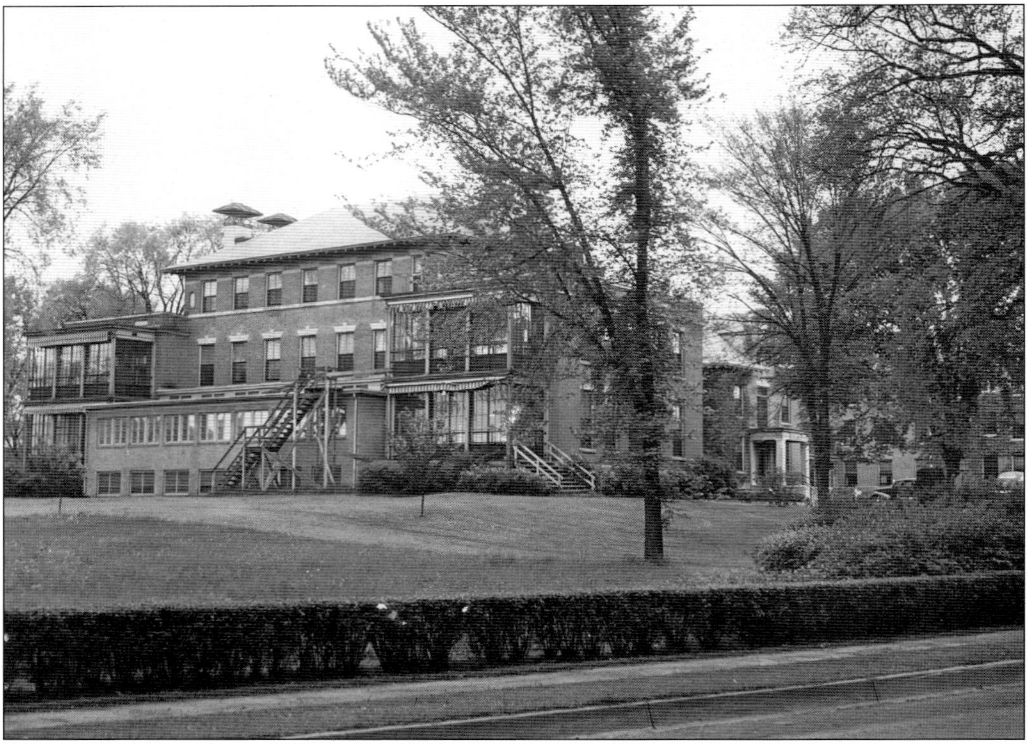

This undated photograph of the South Building reflects the renovations of the original building to enclose the porches and add emergency exit stairways. This view is from High Street, where the current Emergency Department is located. The South Building was demolished after completion of the Spokes in the late 1960s.

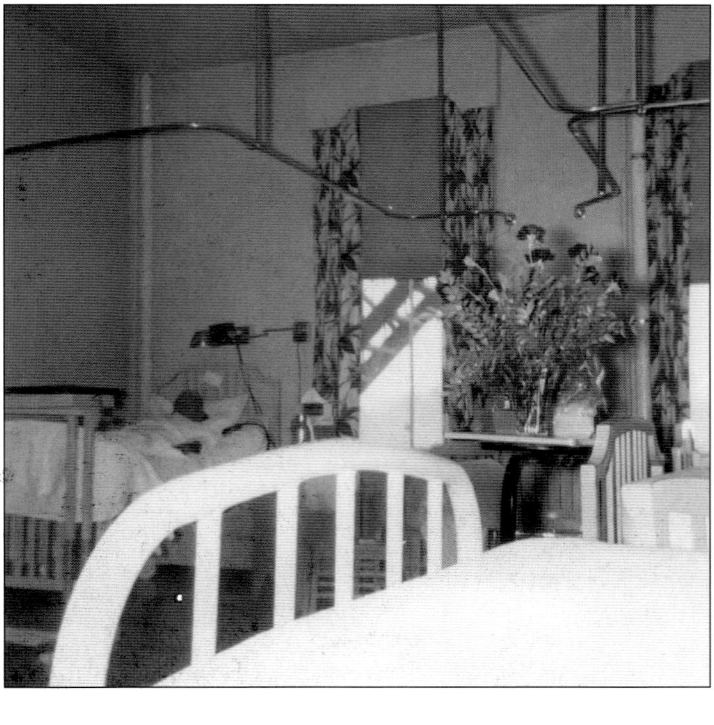

The "old pediatric ward," located in the former porch of the South Building, had been repurposed for adult care by the late 1950s. Note the flowers sitting on a shelf and the rails for the bed curtains around each bed. A note found with this picture reads, "Life can be beautiful even in a ward."

Three

Serving Women and Children

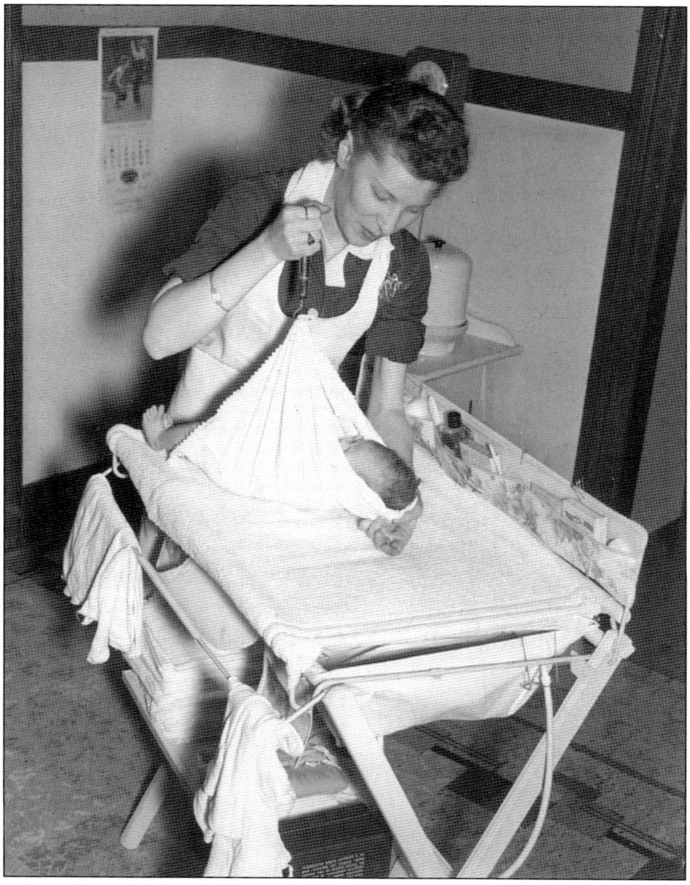

FCPH and the Visiting Nurse Association (VNA) have partnered for almost 120 years. In the mid-1940s, Theresa Bowen, a VNA nurse, weighs a young baby with a hand-held scale. Education has remained an important role for the VNA, particularly for first-time and low-income mothers.

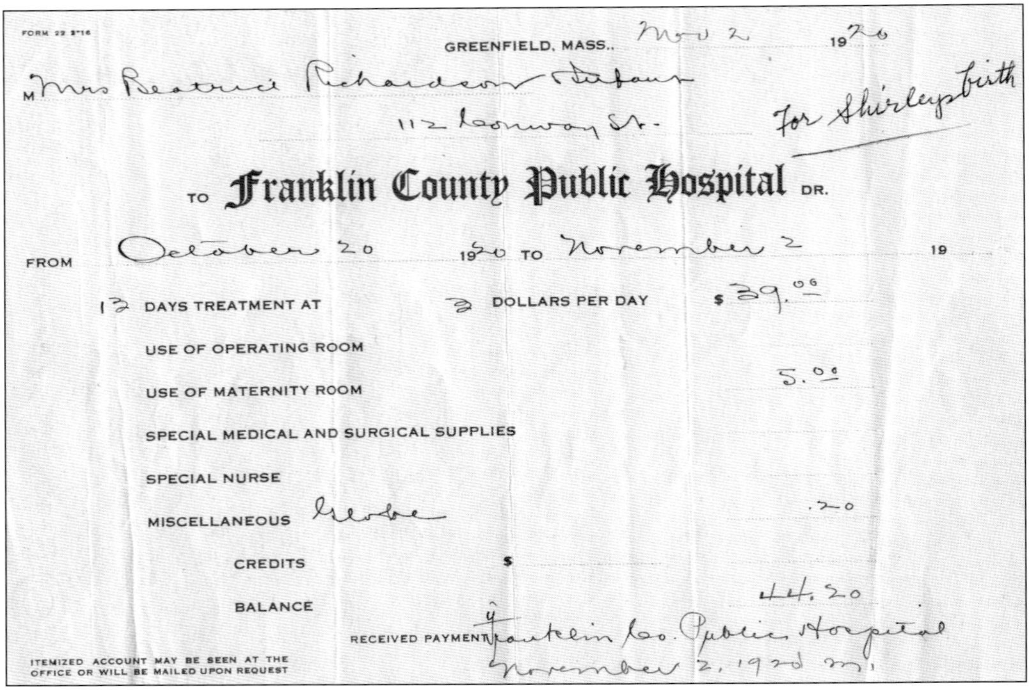

FORM 22 5-16

GREENFIELD, MASS., Nov 2 1920

M Mrs Beatrice Richardson Dufour

112 Conway St.

For Shirley's birth

TO **Franklin County Public Hospital** DR.

FROM October 20 1920 TO November 2 19

13 DAYS TREATMENT AT 3 DOLLARS PER DAY $ 39.00

USE OF OPERATING ROOM

USE OF MATERNITY ROOM 5.00

SPECIAL MEDICAL AND SURGICAL SUPPLIES

SPECIAL NURSE

MISCELLANEOUS Globe .20

CREDITS $

BALANCE 44.20

RECEIVED PAYMENT Franklin Co. Public Hospital November 2, 1920 M.

ITEMIZED ACCOUNT MAY BE SEEN AT THE OFFICE OR WILL BE MAILED UPON REQUEST

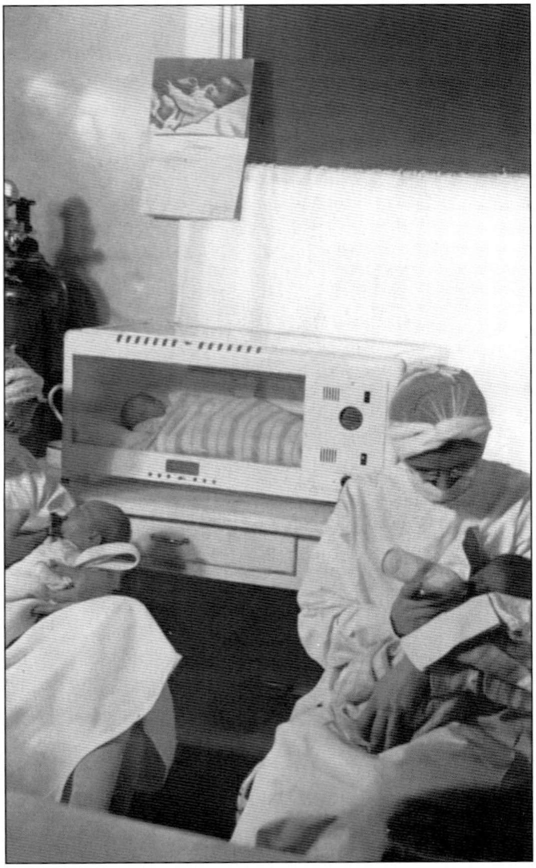

This November 1920 hospital bill shows a maternity inpatient stay of 13 days at the rate of $3 per day along with a $5 charge for the use of the delivery room. The only other expense incurred for the almost two-week admission was 20¢ for gloves. Total cost of the 13-day stay was $44.20. The daily room rate in 2015 for a semi-private maternity room is $1,060 with additional charges for birthing rooms and nursery care, but length of stay is much shorter.

In this 1945 photograph from a fundraising brochure, two nurses bottle-feed infants, with a third baby in an incubator. Maternity cases accounted for about one third of all inpatient hospital visits during the first 100 years of the hospital; between 1925 (the earliest records available) and 1995, 41,000 babies were born at the hospital. BFMC physicians and midwives delivered 497 babies in 2015.

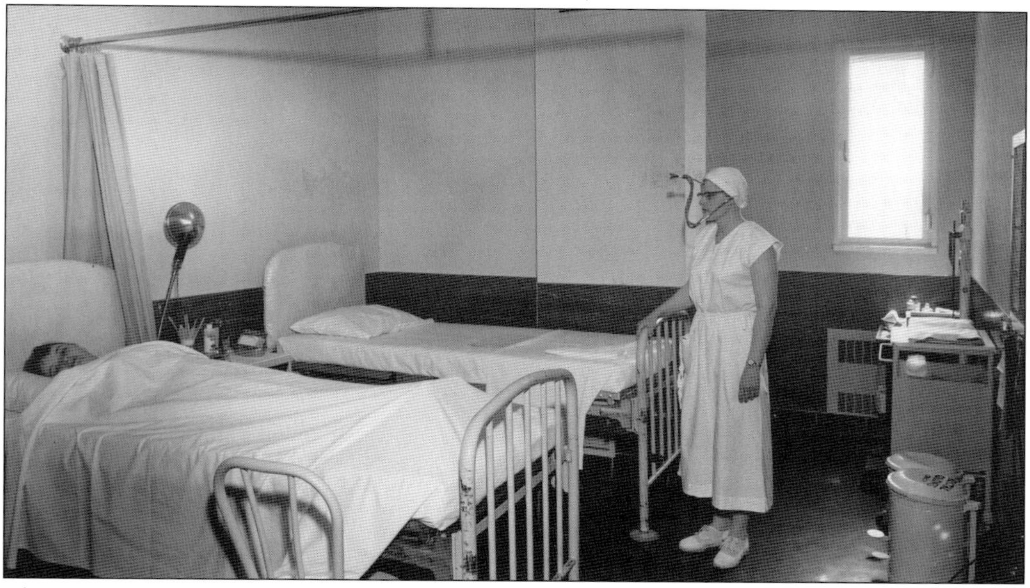

This c. 1950 photograph shows a nurse wearing a fetoscope, a specialized stethoscope that allowed auscultation of the fetal heart rate while leaving the nurse's or obstetrician's hands free to position the mother's uterus. In the days before electronic fetal heart monitors or ultrasound machines, these devices monitored the health of the baby prior to delivery. Today, the term fetoscope refers to a fiber-optic device allowing direct visualization. The hand-cranked beds are long gone. The average number of mother-and-child patients was 14 per day in 1927 and increased to 36 per day in 1945.

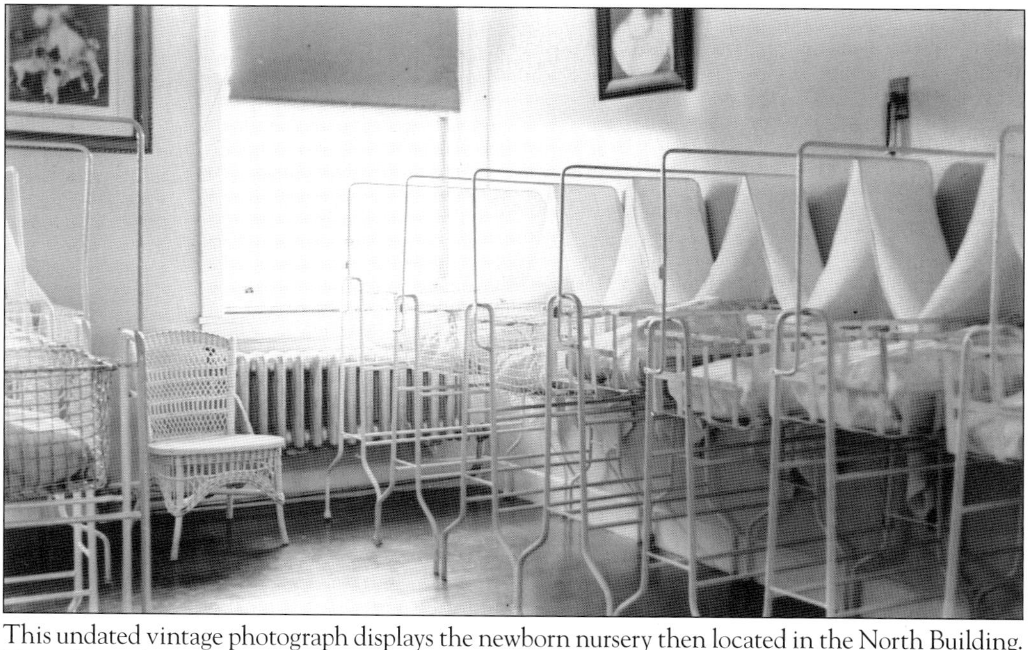

This undated vintage photograph displays the newborn nursery then located in the North Building. Note the wicker chairs and the bassinets equipped with fabric tenting, both of which would be banned under modern infection control. From 1944 to 1950, the number of babies born at FCPH increased from 556 to 743, marking the onset of the Baby Boom. Another "boomlet" occurred between 1968 and 1970, when the number of newborns increased from 555 to 706.

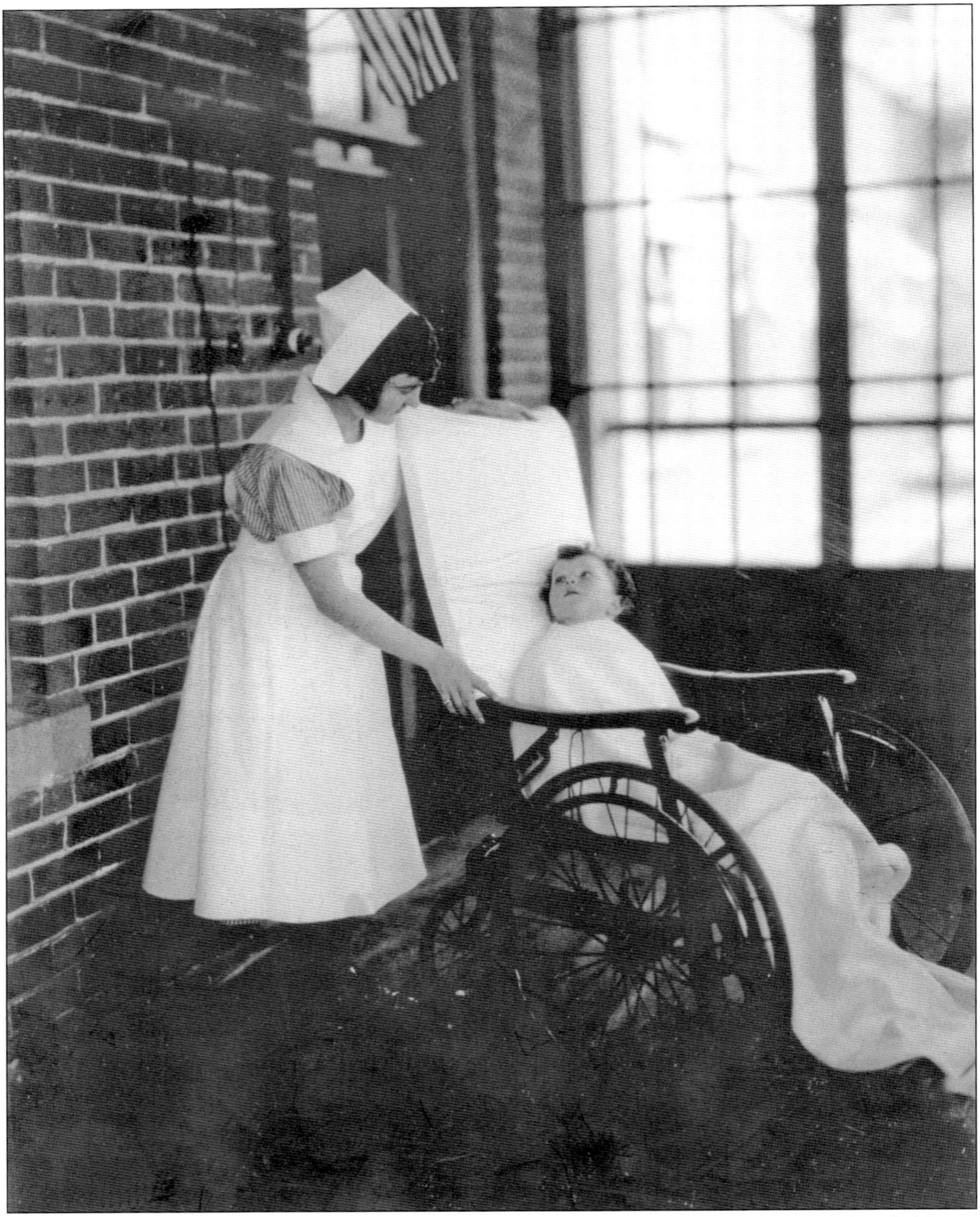

In this 1934 photograph, a student nurse adjusts the wheelchair for a patient in the children's ward. A similar photograph appeared in a fundraising advertisement in the *Greenfield Recorder* on May 18, 1934. The fundraising took place to raise $65,000 to retire an accumulated deficit due to charity work at the hospital.

VNA nurse Theresa Bowen gives a newborn baby a sponge bath in the mid-1940s. The VNA, then as now, brings medical services and education to homes in the community.

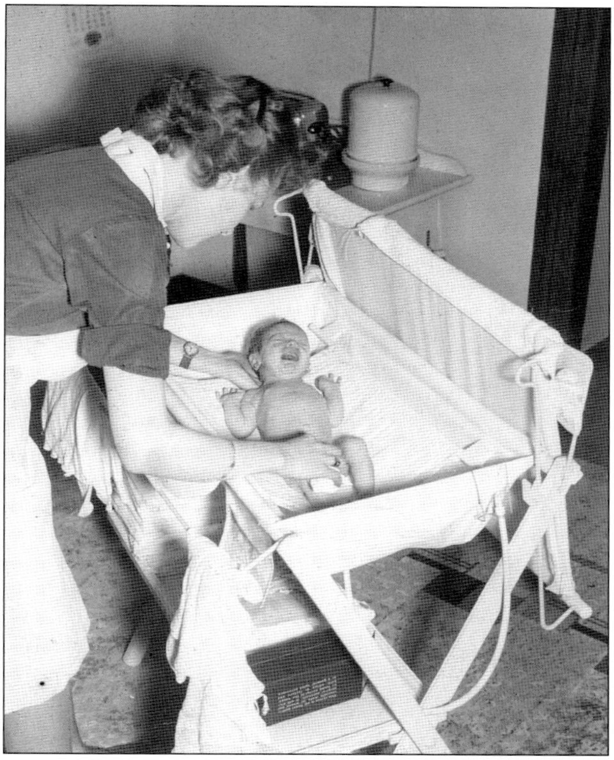

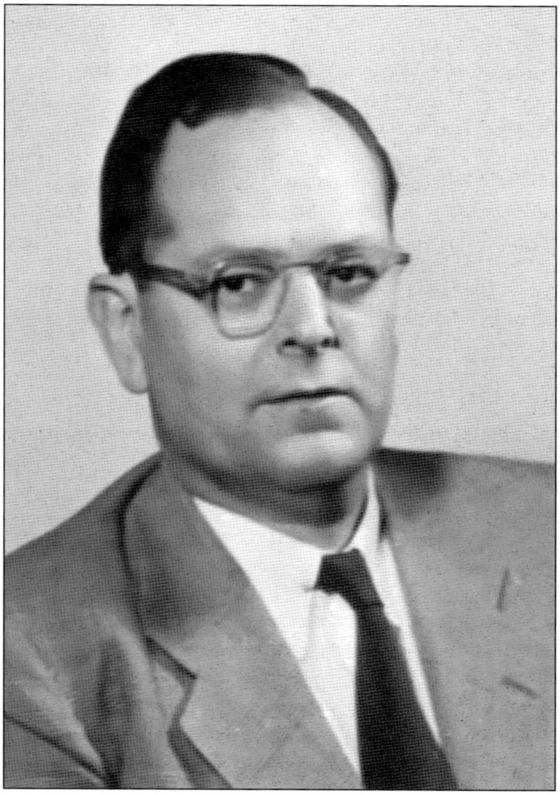

Dr. Merritt Low was a beloved pediatrician in Franklin County for 48 years, having cared for thousands of infants and children. He was the first pediatrician in the county; he set up his practice in 1937 and opened the FCPH clinic for the children of the poor. In 1943, while caring for his young patients, he contracted polio, which he felt lucky to survive, but not without becoming crippled, needing to use crutches and a wheelchair for the remainder of his life. Dr. Low became president of the American Academy of Pediatrics in 1975 and a passionate advocate for care of the disabled.

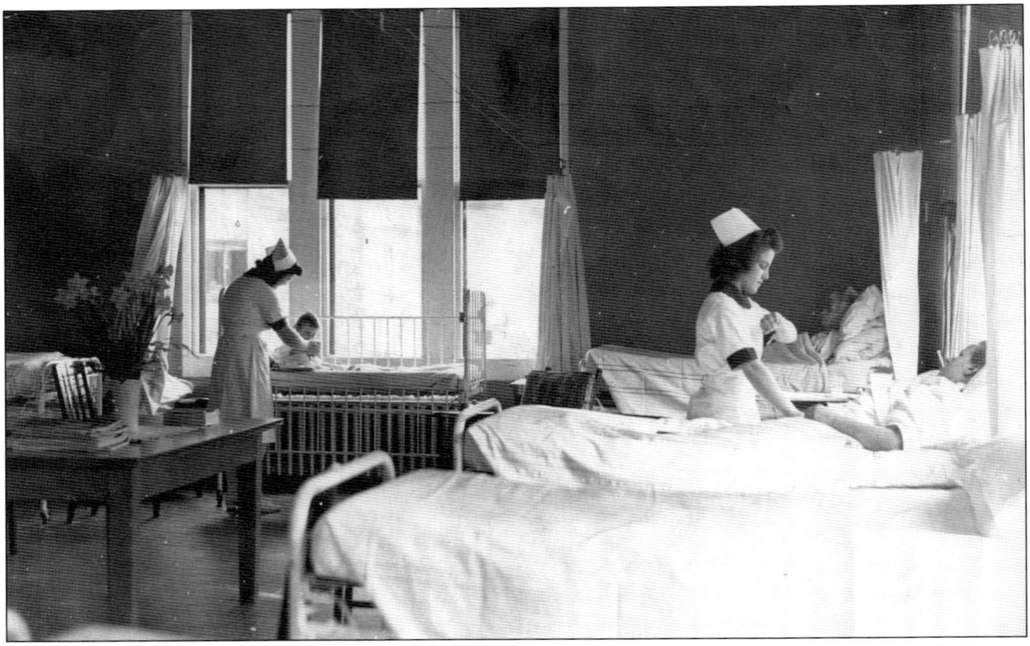

Student nurses are making their rounds on the 1 South open ward. The presence of a child in a crib under the windows suggests this was before a separate pediatric ward was created from the former porch on 1 South. The daffodils on the table suggest this photograph was taken in the spring, likely in the 1940s.

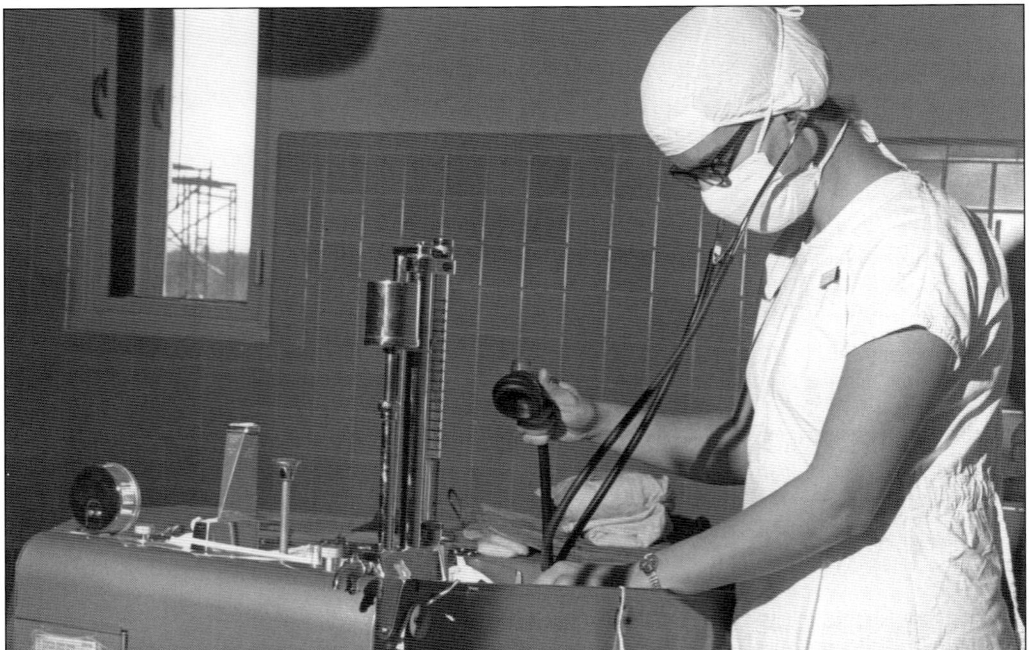

Cecilia C. "CeeCee" Sherman, RN, is pictured with a Kreiselman infant resuscitator; one was located in every delivery room. This equipment was used to initiate respiration in newborn babies who had difficulty breathing. CeeCee worked at FCPH/BFMC from 1974 to 2005, only briefly as a registered nurse in obstetrics and the remaining years as an emergency room nurse.

Current BFMC employees Sue (Whitney) LaCoy, left, a three-year employee, and Sandy (Whitney) Campbell, right, a 14-year employee, were approximately six months old at the time of this photograph. They were the first set of twins born at FCPH in 1959. Their mother, Phyllis Whitney, was also an employee of FCPH from 1971 through 1983, making the hospital a family affair for this Franklin County family. (Courtesy of Sue LaCoy.)

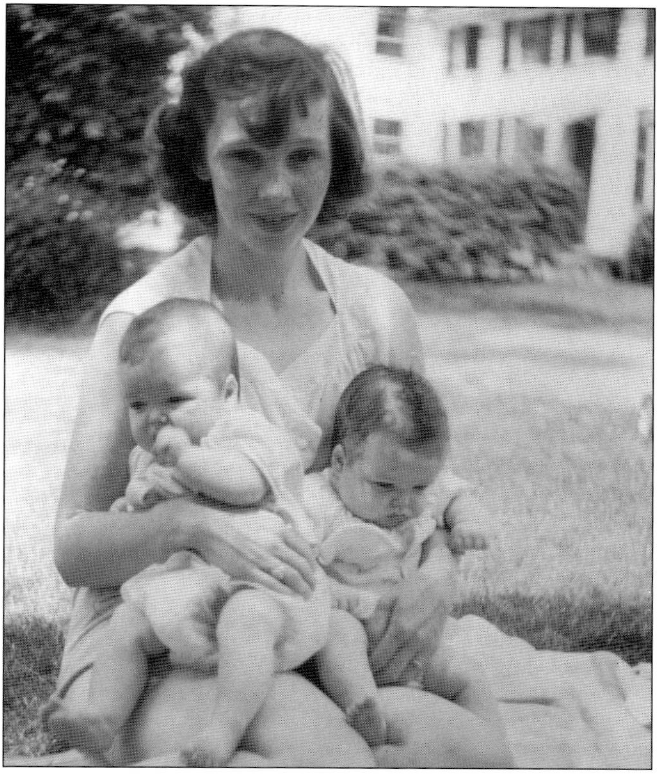

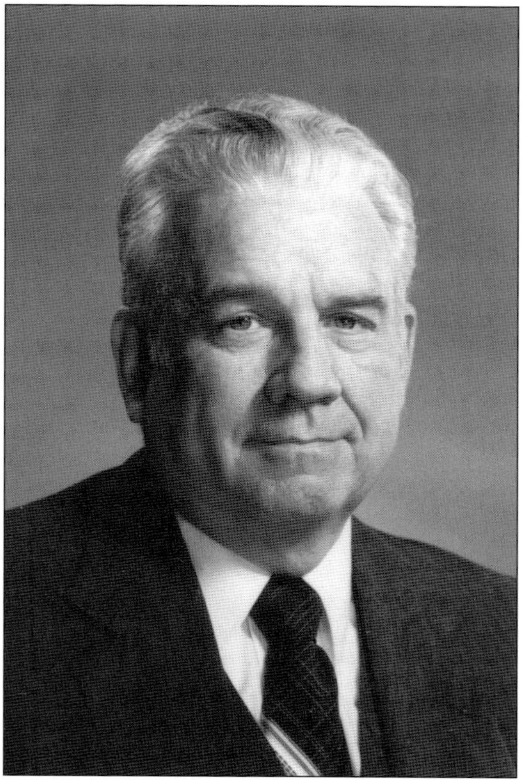

Dr. Percy Wadman was an obstetrician-gynecologist at FCPH from 1955 to 1986, moving to Baystate Medical Center until retiring in 1998. He was one of four FCPH/BFMC physicians who served as Massachusetts Medical Society (MMS) president, serving in 1982. His portrait hangs today in the Percy Wadman Boardroom at the MMS headquarters in Waltham.

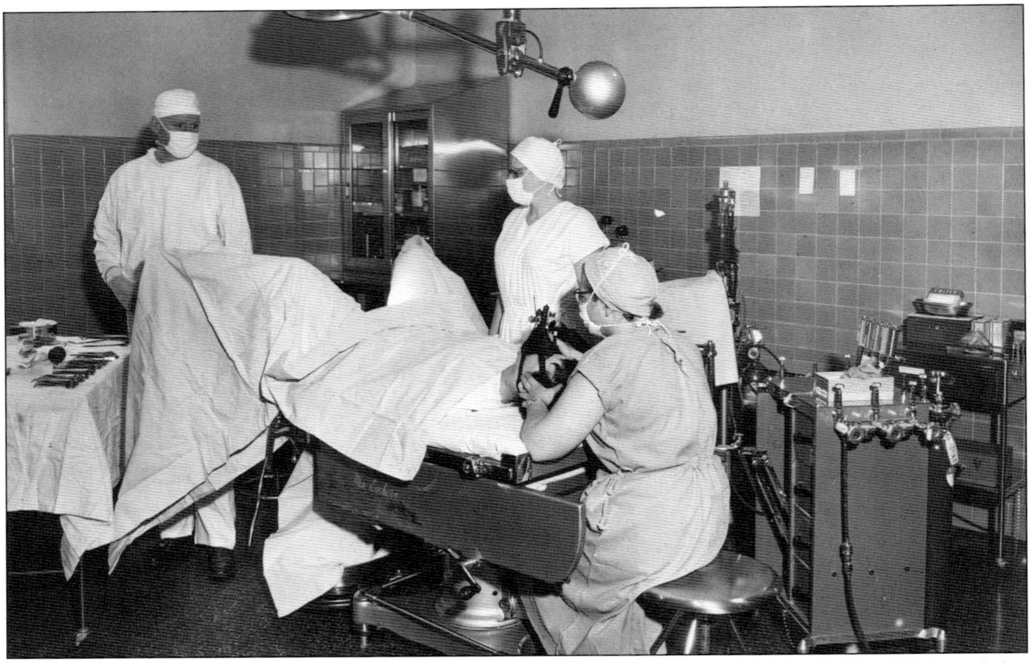

A delivery is in progress around 1974 in one of the delivery rooms on the third floor of the Central Building. The patient is receiving inhalational anesthetic through a black mask that is stabilized to her face with head straps. The obstetrician, circulating nurse, and nurse anesthetist are unidentified.

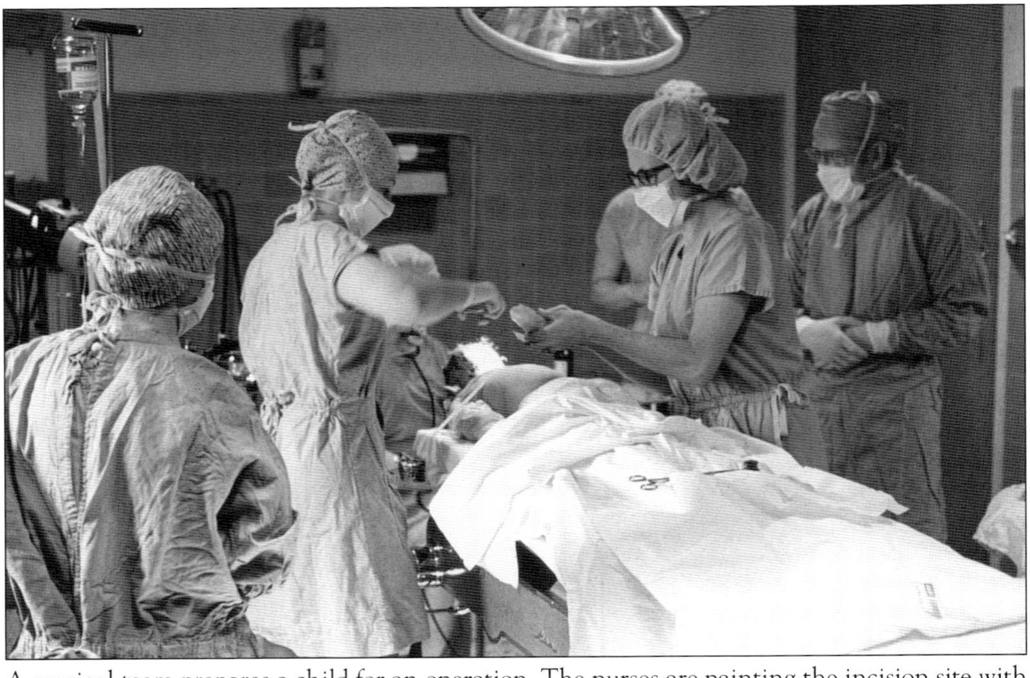

A surgical team prepares a child for an operation. The nurses are painting the incision site with topical antiseptic while the gloved and gowned surgeon, carefully holding his arms in to preserve sterility, watches from the right. This photograph was taken in the old operating room on 2 North in 1974.

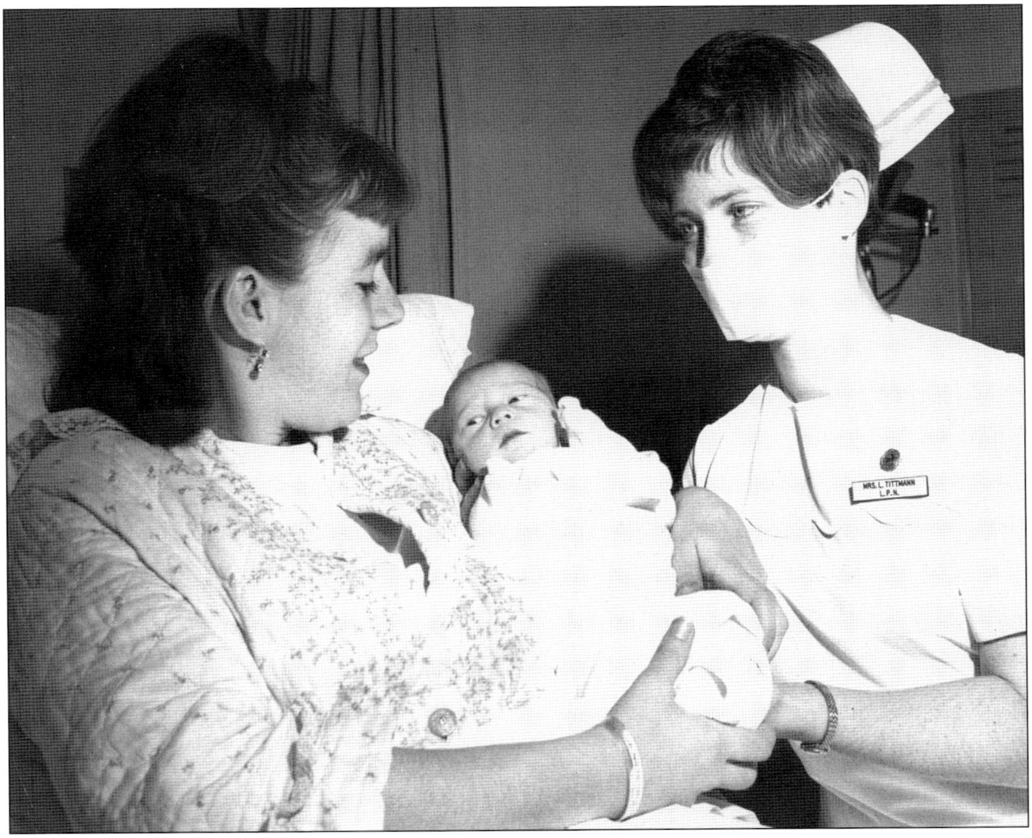

FCPH has always had an active maternity service, growing from a handful of deliveries at the hospital's inception to nearly 500 per year today. In this 1968 photograph, Carol Reed and her infant daughter are tended to by Laureen Tittmann, LPN.

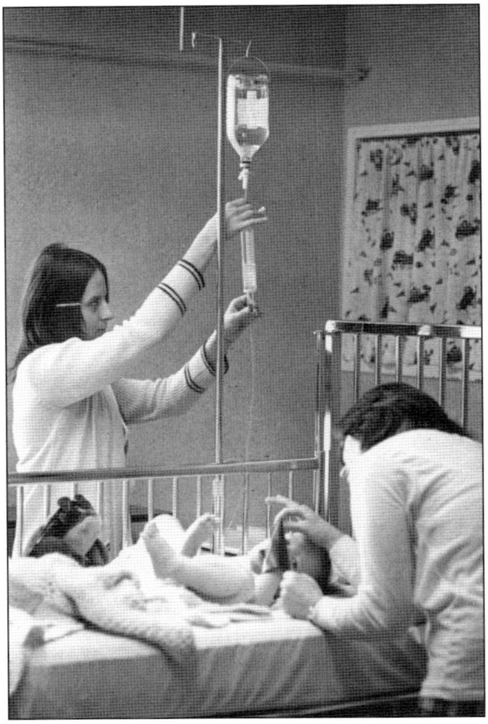

Diane Witkos, RN, adjusts the IV of a pediatric patient in 1975. The pediatric unit was located in Spoke 2 at that time. From 1974 to 1992, Witkos was a pediatric nurse; in 2015, she is still employed by Baystate Health as a clinical informatics analyst.

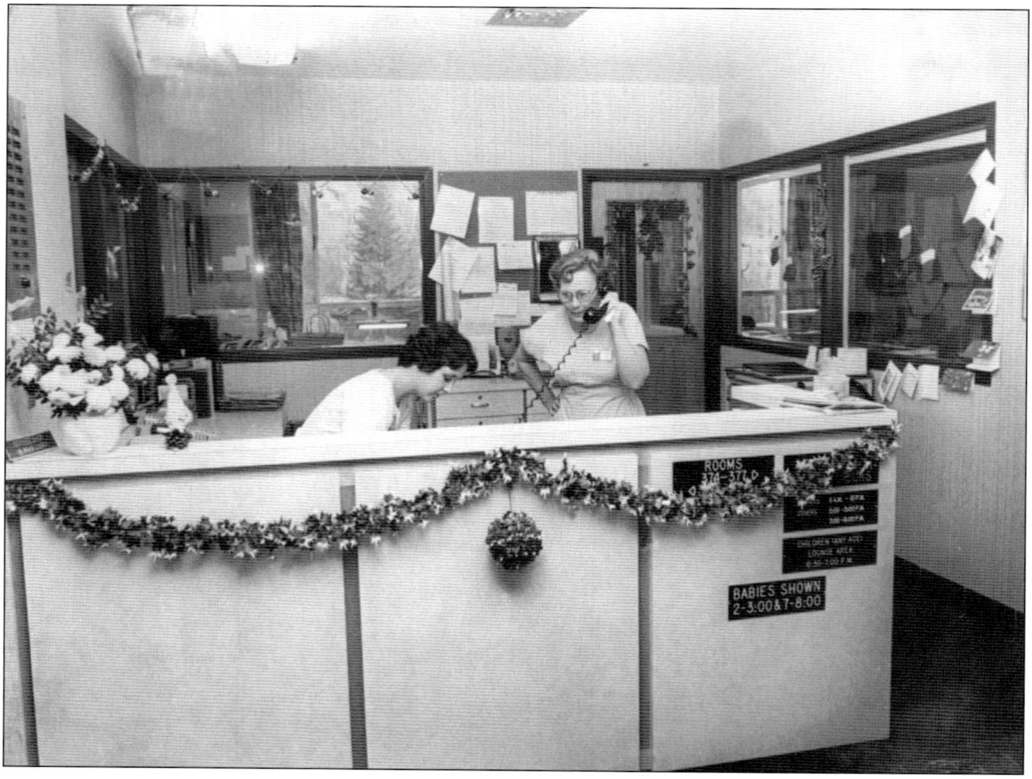

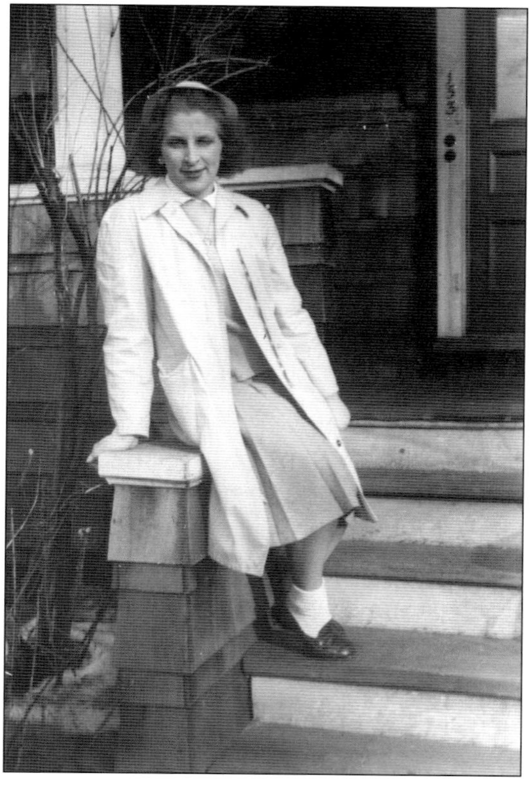

The nursing station on the third floor obstetrics ward is decorated for the holidays in this c. 1970s photograph. Nurse Frances Griffin is on the telephone, while Chris Beaulieu is busy doing paperwork. Note the limited times posted that babies could be viewed in the glassed-in rooms located to the sides of the nursing station. Visiting rules would be relaxed shortly after with the advent of the Birthplace.

A member of the FCPH School of Nursing class of 1945, Dorothy "Dottie" Jennis Telega is pictured here. She was a supervisor, then manager, in the OB/GYN department and worked her entire career at FCPH/FMC until she passed away in 1993.

This 1980 photograph of Dottie Telega, RN, along with a new mother and infant, was taken in her later years as nursing supervisor. She was behind the initiation of the birthing center, now known as the Birthplace at BFMC. She also was responsible for bringing the use of birthing rooms to the hospital and supported Susan Liddell, CNM, in the introduction of birthing bath tubs for water births as alternatives for women who delivered their children at BFMC.

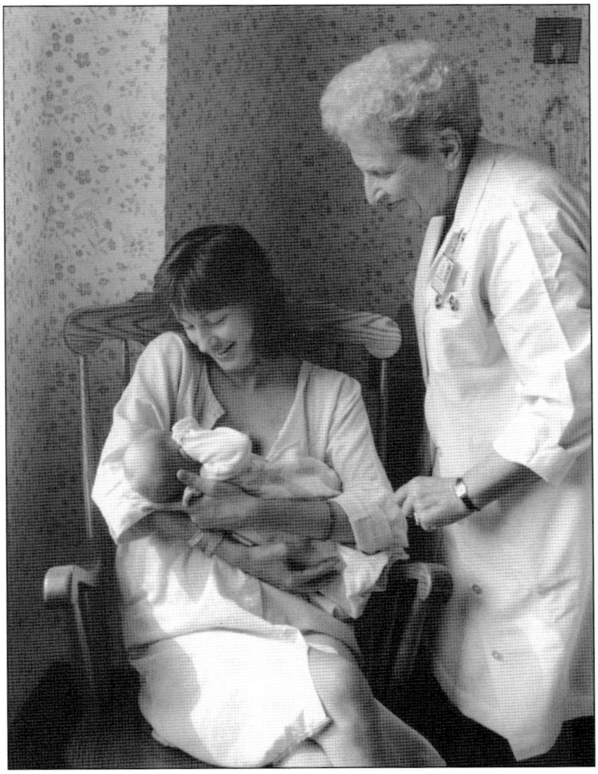

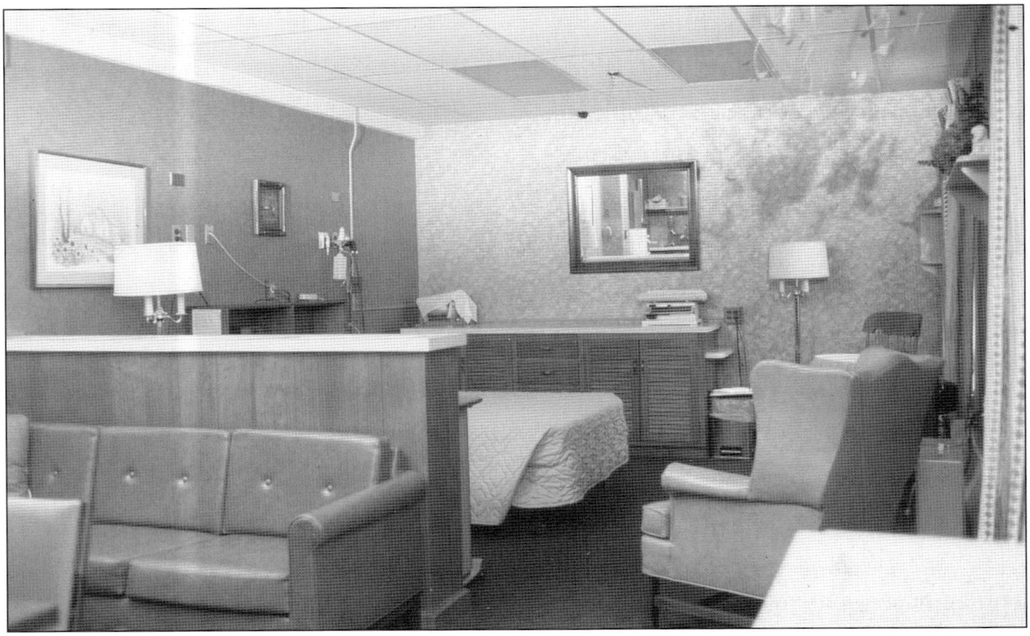

Pictured around the late 1980s is one of the first birthing rooms available for delivering babies. This room provided a more home-like atmosphere with a standard double bed instead of a hospital bed. The setup also allowed the mother to both labor and deliver in the same room, instead of having to be moved to the delivery room. The father (or labor partner) was also able to stay overnight with the mother, and other family members were allowed in the room as well.

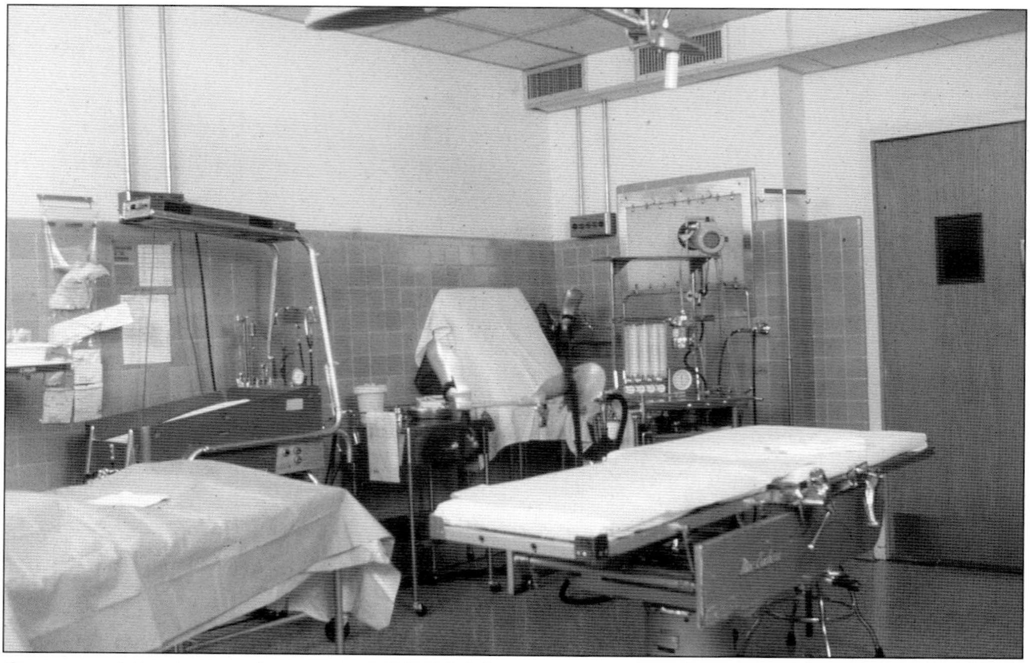

Compare this picture of a standard FCPH delivery room around 1980 with the previous image. While this stark environment is much less welcoming than the birthing room, patients could be reassured that technology such as the incubator at left and the operating table and anesthesia equipment at right were readily available down the hall if needed.

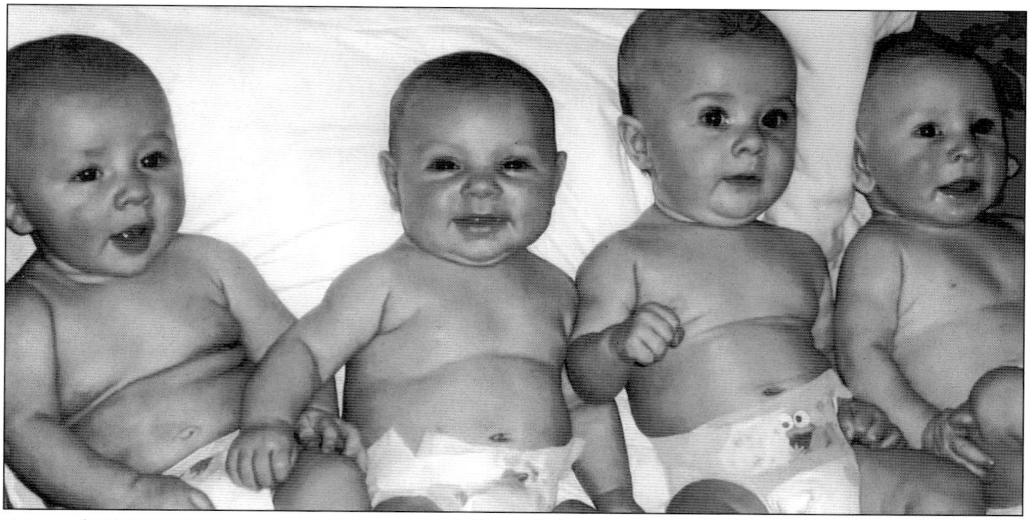

Around 2005, infant massage "classmates" (from left to right, Atticus Peters, Meredith Bedell, Elias Lundquist, and Ben Tardif) were featured in a local advertisement for The Birthplace at Baystate Franklin.

Four

The FCPH School of Nursing

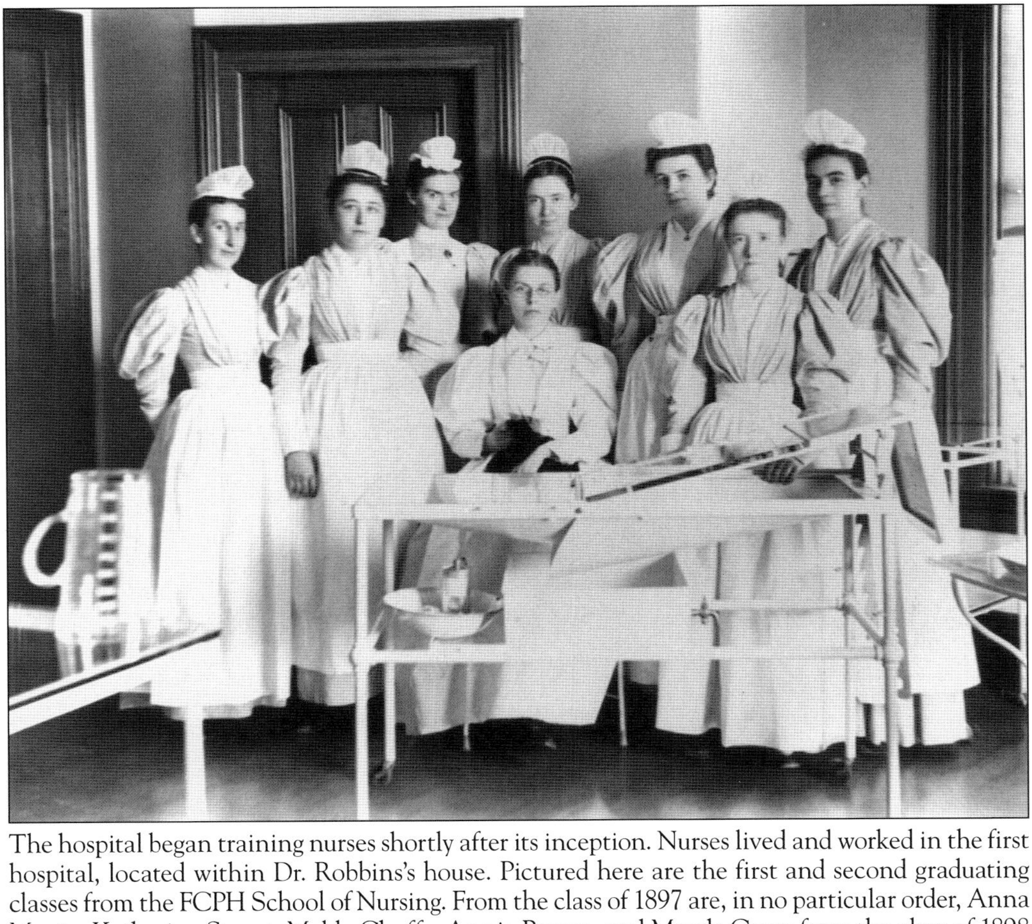

The hospital began training nurses shortly after its inception. Nurses lived and worked in the first hospital, located within Dr. Robbins's house. Pictured here are the first and second graduating classes from the FCPH School of Nursing. From the class of 1897 are, in no particular order, Anna Moritz, Katherine Stuart, Mable Chaffe, Annie Brown, and Maude Gour; from the class of 1898 are Grace Page, Katherine Martin, Mary Conroy, and Emily Young.

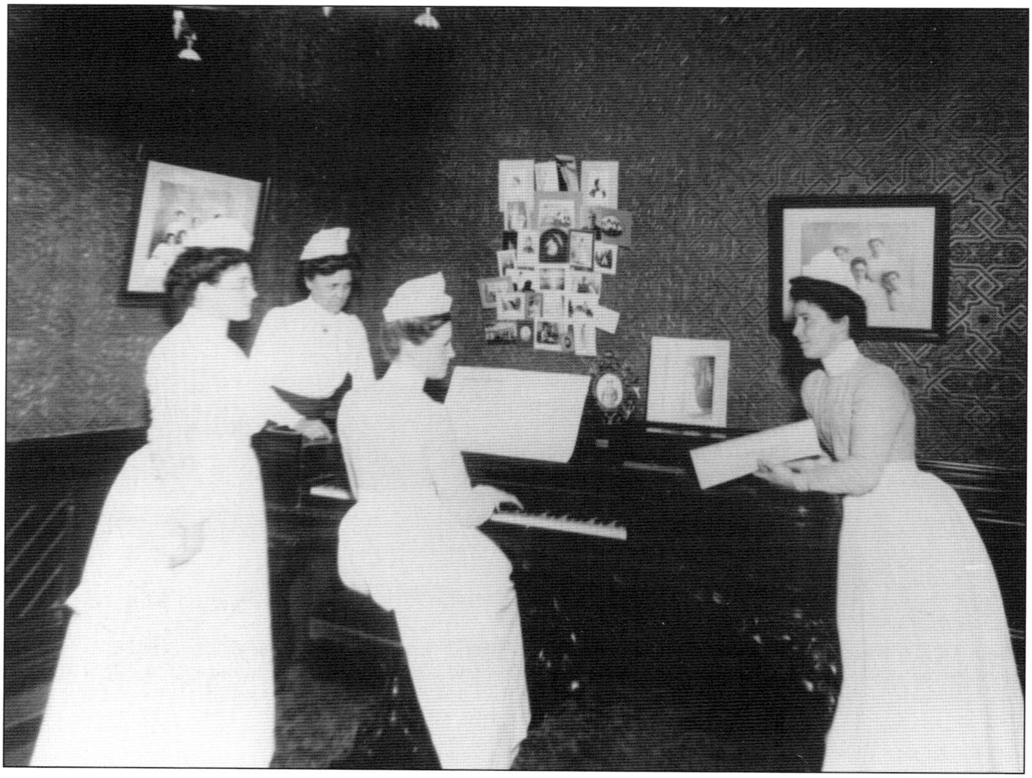

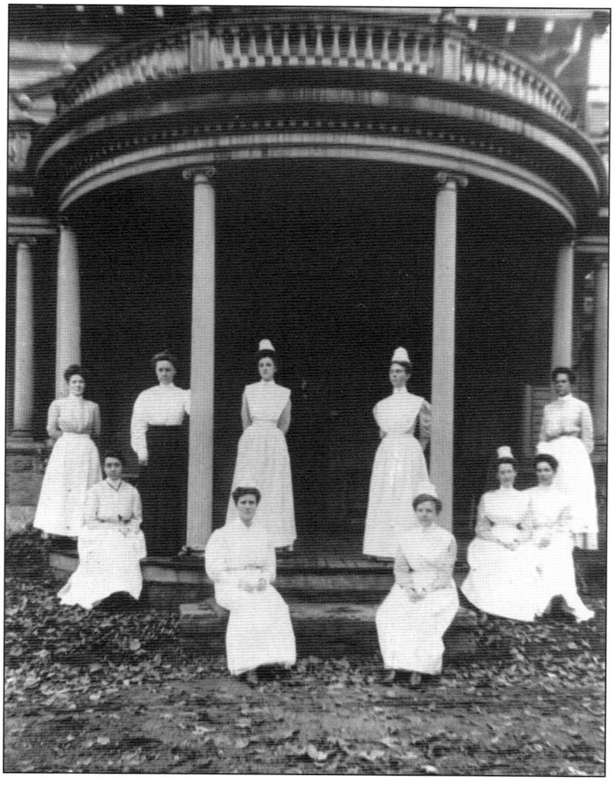

The nurses' quarters were located on the top floor of the hospital's second location in the Converse House, used from 1898 to 1910. In this 1903 photograph, nursing students gather around the piano. Behind the piano is Anna M. Sweeney, the superintendent. Ethel McLean is playing.

The graduates of the FCPH School of Nursing classes of 1906, 1907, and 1908 are seated on the porch of the second location of the FCPH on the corner of Main and Conway Streets. The hospital would soon move to a new facility on High Street.

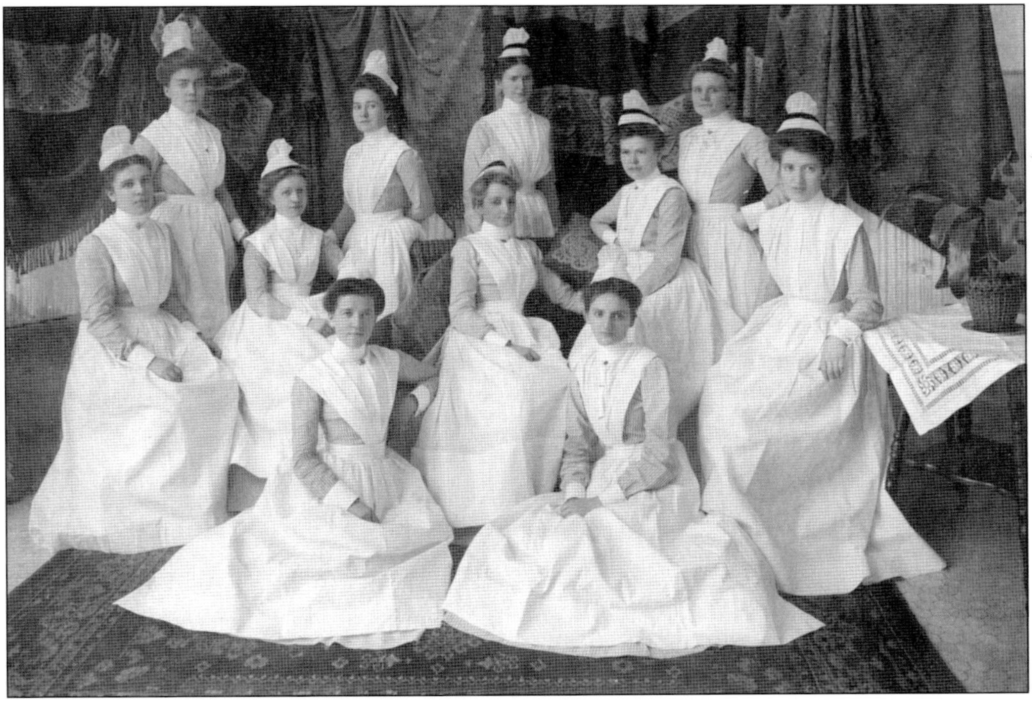

Pictured is the FCPH School of Nursing class of 1902. Among the graduates was Anna Koch, who was to become a leader in social justice and mental health. Early in her career, she worked with Reverend Whiteman and others to create the local Visiting Nurses Association (VNA) in 1910. Koch was the sole employee of the VNA in 1911, where she saw 112 patients in 970 home visits.

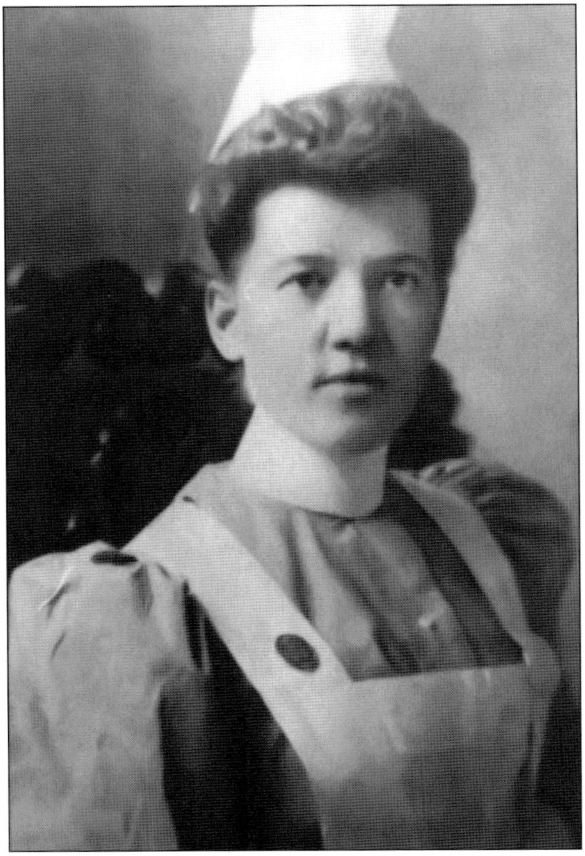

Anna Koch, RN, was the daughter of German parents. After forming the VNA in 1910, she formed the Society for Prevention of Cruelty to Children in 1914 and the Well Baby Clinic in 1920, and later worked with Drs. Merritt Low and Lawrence Dame to create Greenfield's first mental health center.

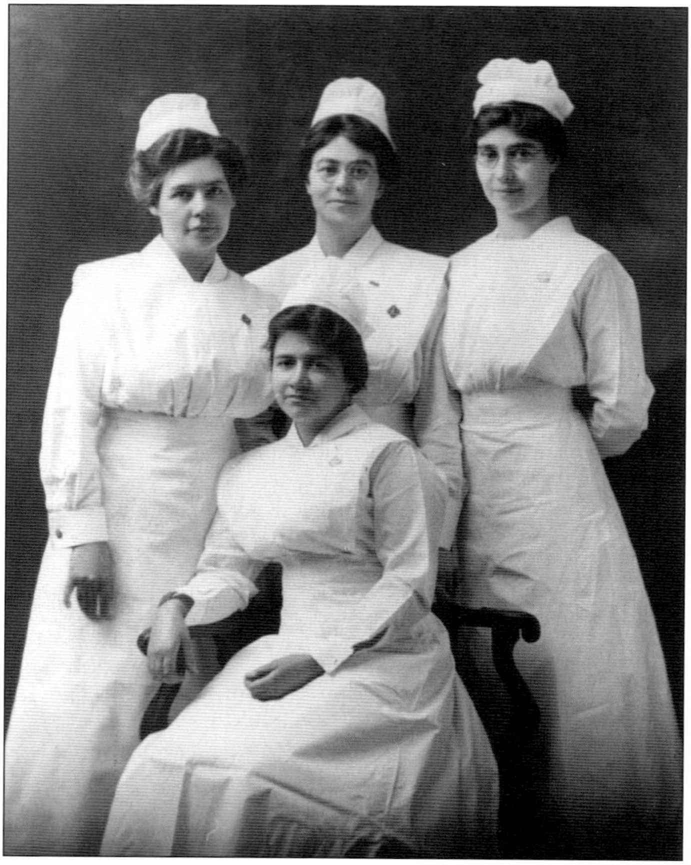

Four of the seven graduates of the FCPH School of Nursing class of 1912 are shown here. Upon graduation, nurses in the early years were given a diploma, a class pin, and $50. Pictured are Marjorie Robertson, Annabelle Mackenzie (Stetson), and Anna MacDonald. (Courtesy of Greenfield Community College.)

Pictured here is the FCPH School of Nursing class of 1913. Note that each graduate has her diploma in hand, beautifully tied with a bow. From left to right are (seated) Laura Dawson Morrel, superintendent Anna Sweeney, and two unidentified; (standing) Alice Cain Holland, Mabel Thompson Brown, Elizabeth Dorgan Davis, Mable Cooper Mack, and Katherine Mackenzie Holmes.

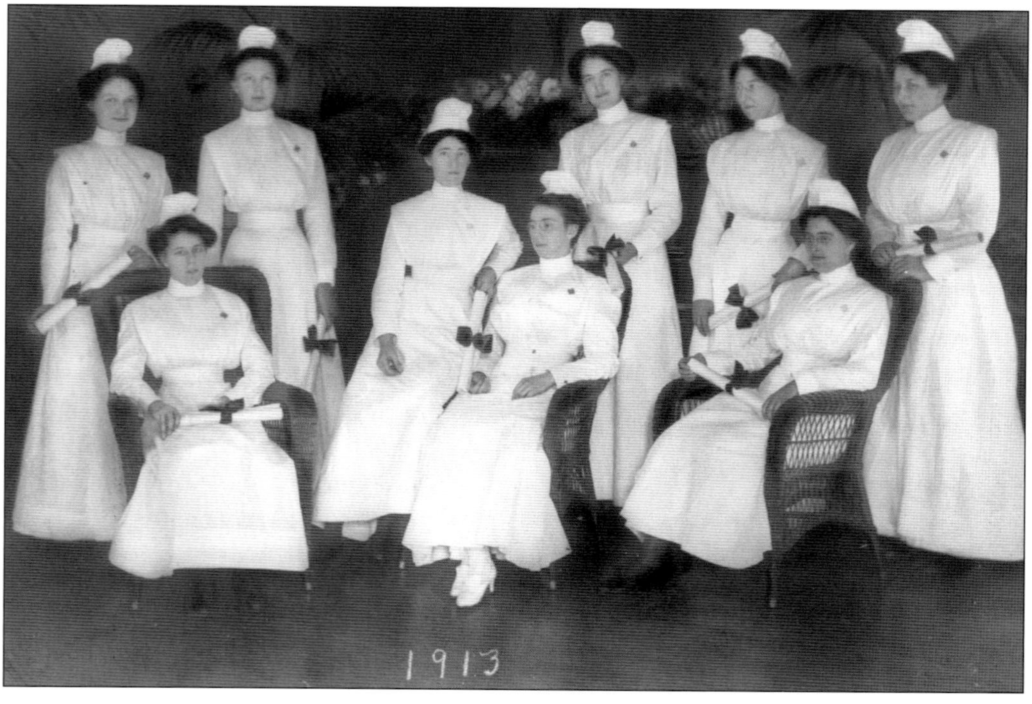

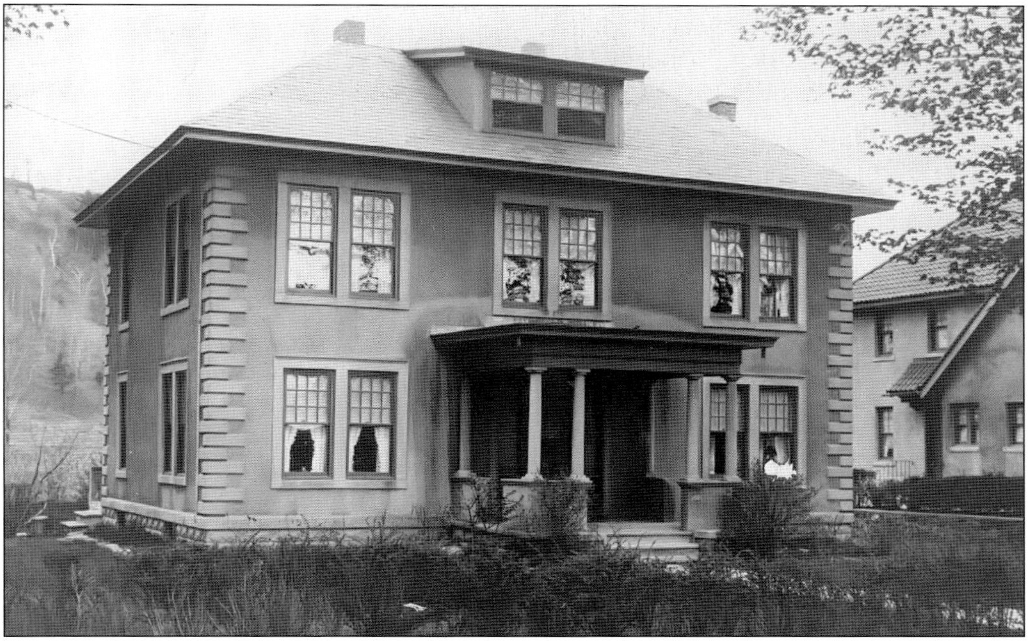

In 1915, the Franklin County Public Hospital purchased a house at the corner of Beacon and High Streets to use as a nurses' home. This nursing residence was in use until 1927. Today, the house is a private residence across from the present-day hospital on High Street.

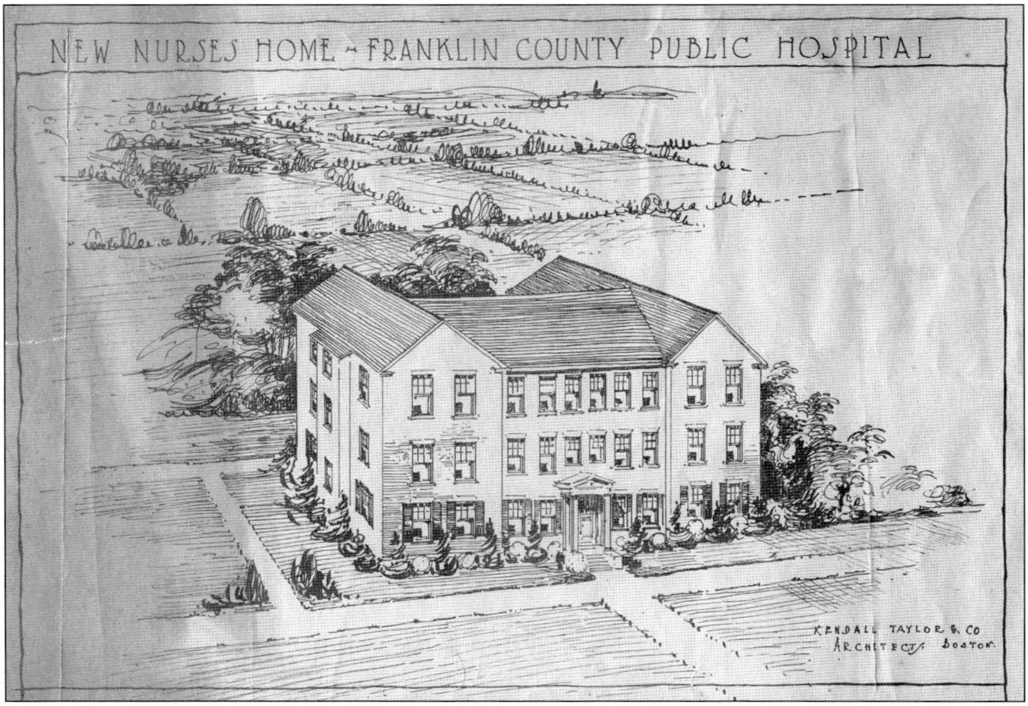

In 1925, a fund drive was held to raise money for a new nurses' home, which was completed in 1927. An artist's sketch of the building is shown here. The building was located adjacent to the main hospital building and later became the Medical Office Building. It was torn down around 2010 in preparation for the new surgery center, scheduled to open in 2016.

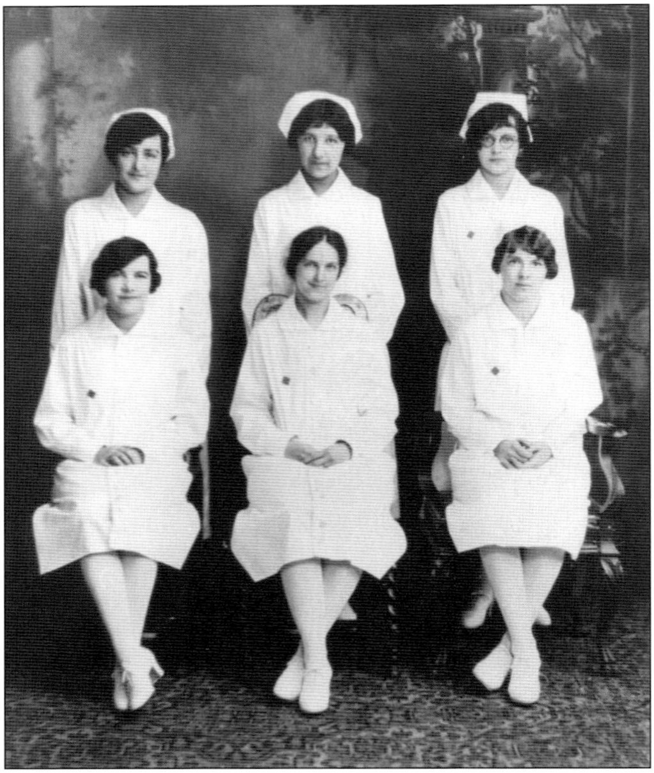

The graduates of the FCPH School of Nursing class of 1927 are (first row) Hazel Davenport, Laura Eastman, and Catherine Egan; (second row) Eleanor Smith, Susie Walking Bear, and Doris Greenway. Susie Walking Bear was the first Native American to become a registered nurse. After graduating from the nursing school, she married Tom Yellowtail and practiced nursing on the Crow Reservation.

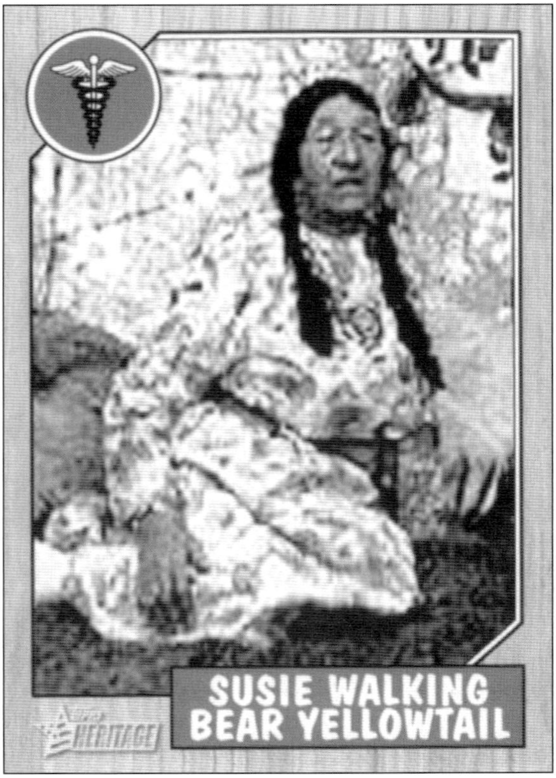

Susie Walking Bear Yellowtail later took a position with the Indian Health Service and from 1930 to 1960 traveled to reservations throughout America, working to address health, social, and education problems for Native Americans. She was the founder of the Native American Nurses Association and was instrumental in securing financial support for Native Americans to become registered nurses. Her contributions to nursing were noted with this bubblegum card. (TLH.)

This is the FCPH School of Nursing class of 1928. Note the change in uniform to a dress that falls below the knee but not to the floor, as seen in 1913. As was tradition, the nursing school provided its graduates with a pin and cap. Pictured are Lois Haskell, Helen Walker, Emily Hamilton, and Helen Thurston.

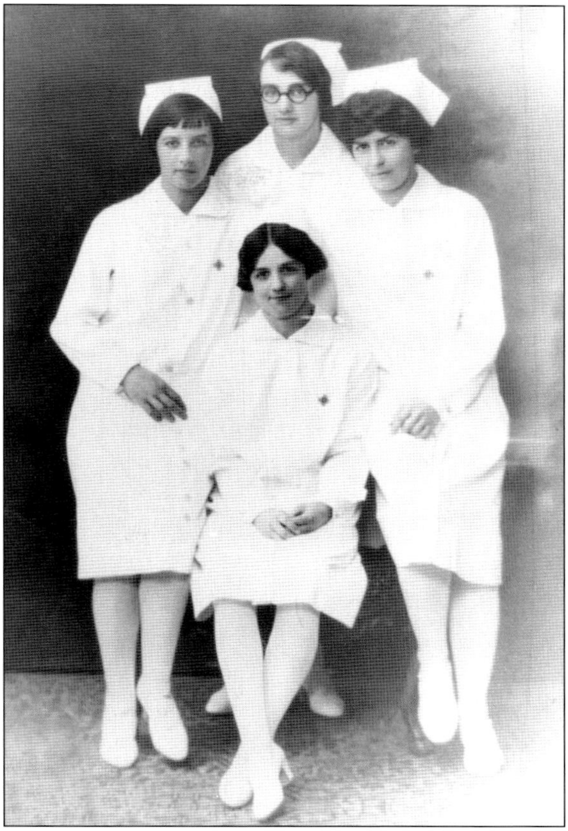

These graduates of the FCPH School of Nursing class of 1934 are Helen Soper, Mildred Call, Helen Start, Minnie Block, Dorothy Tolson, Gertrude March, and Thelma Tatham.

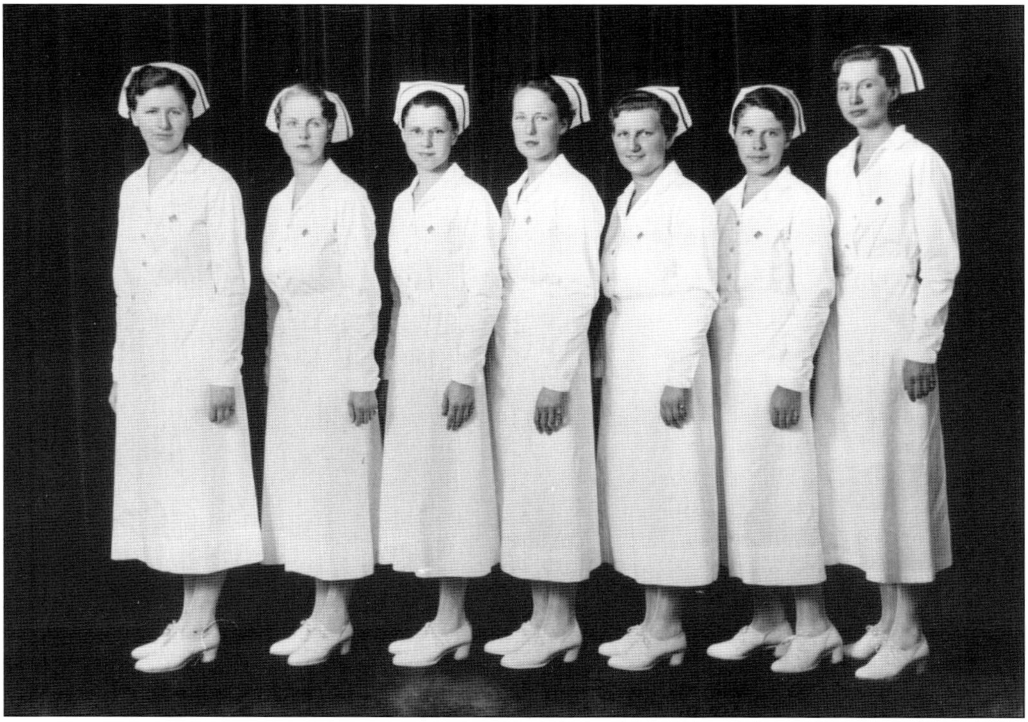

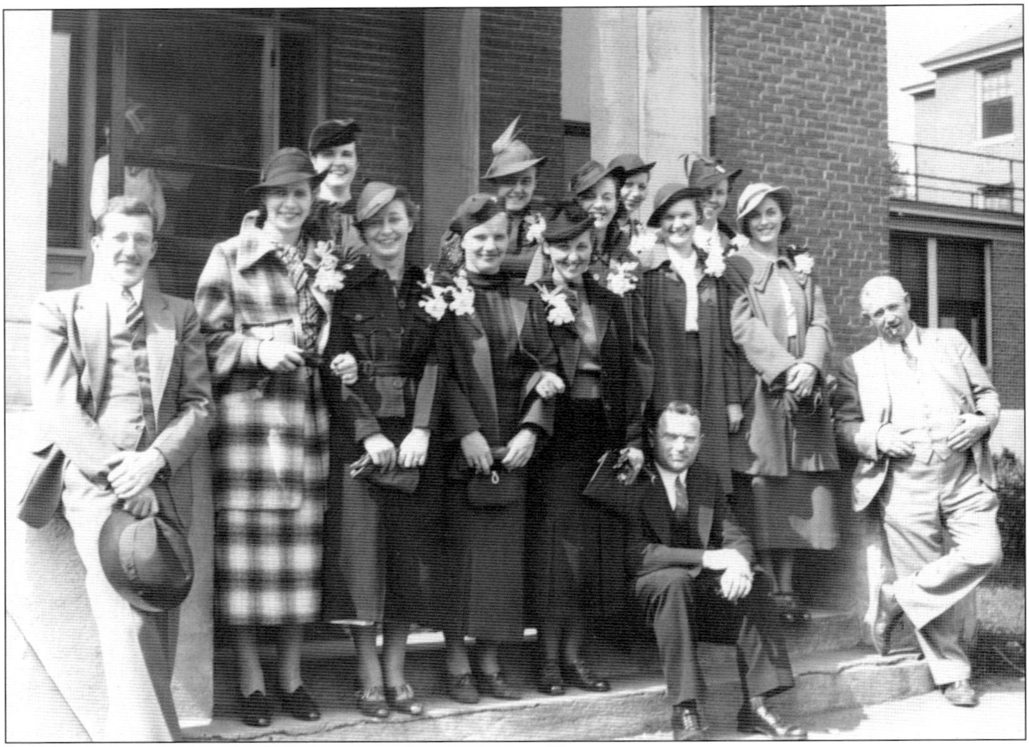

Pictured here is the FCPH School of Nursing class of 1936. In contrast to previous images of the graduates standing stiffly in their starched whites, the class of 1936 posed for this less formal photograph on the steps of the Administration Building. Pictured with the graduates are Dr. Chauncey W. Percy (far left), Dr. Arthur H. Ellis (far right), and an unidentified man seated on the steps.

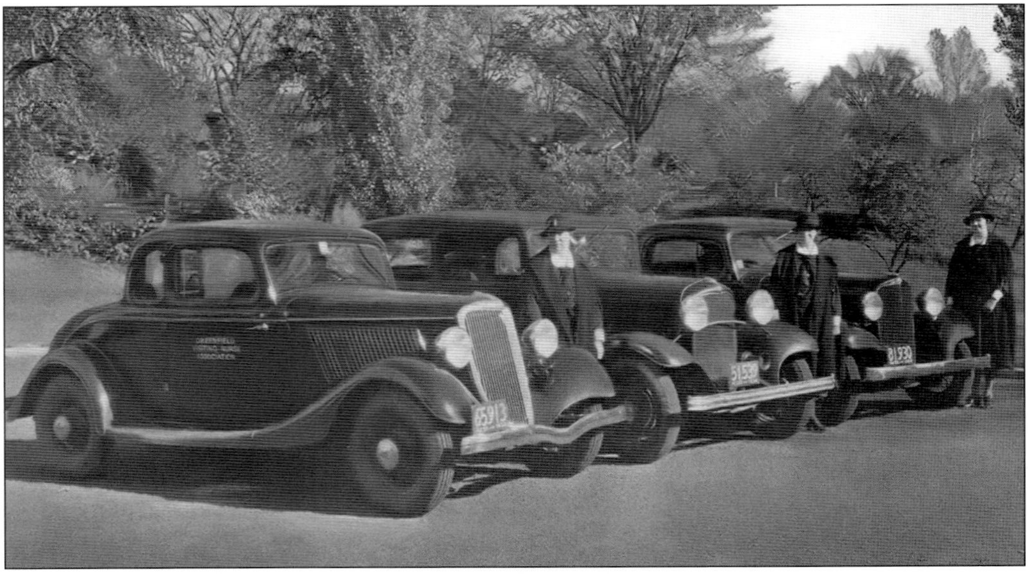

Three nurses from the Greenfield VNA pose alongside their vehicles around 1938.

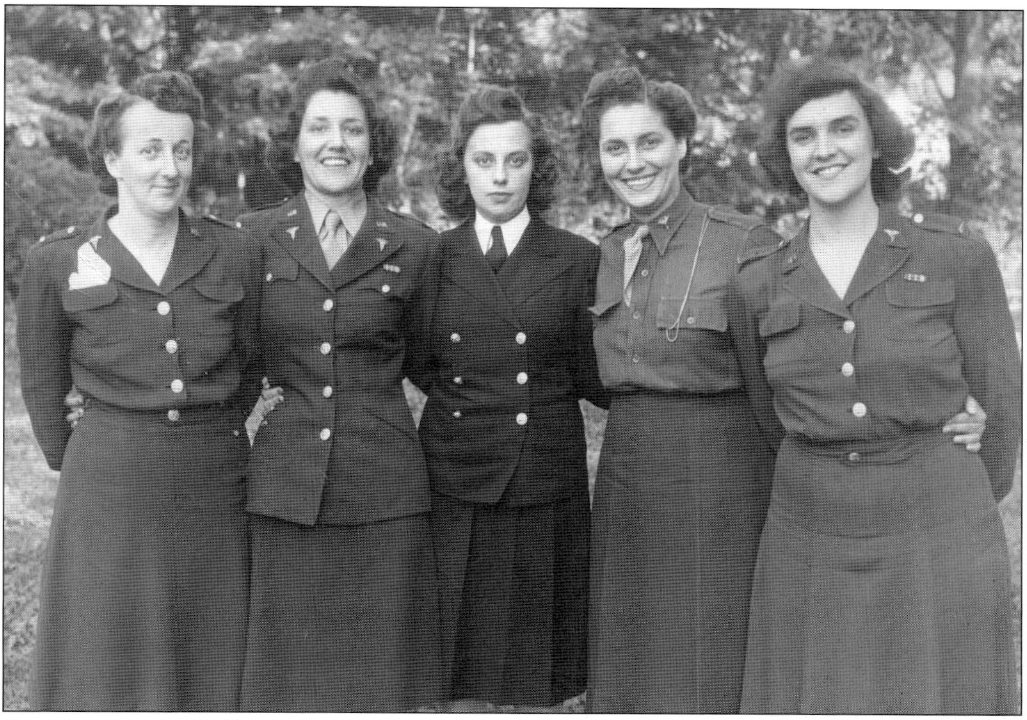

Franklin County Public Hospital nurses served in World War II. Pictured are Grace Ellis Baker, Marge LaPalme Fritz, Marge Twyon Rivard, Dorothy Tullio, and Helen LaPalme Fritz. Marge and Helen LaPalme Fritz are sisters. Note the styles of uniforms representing different branches of the services.

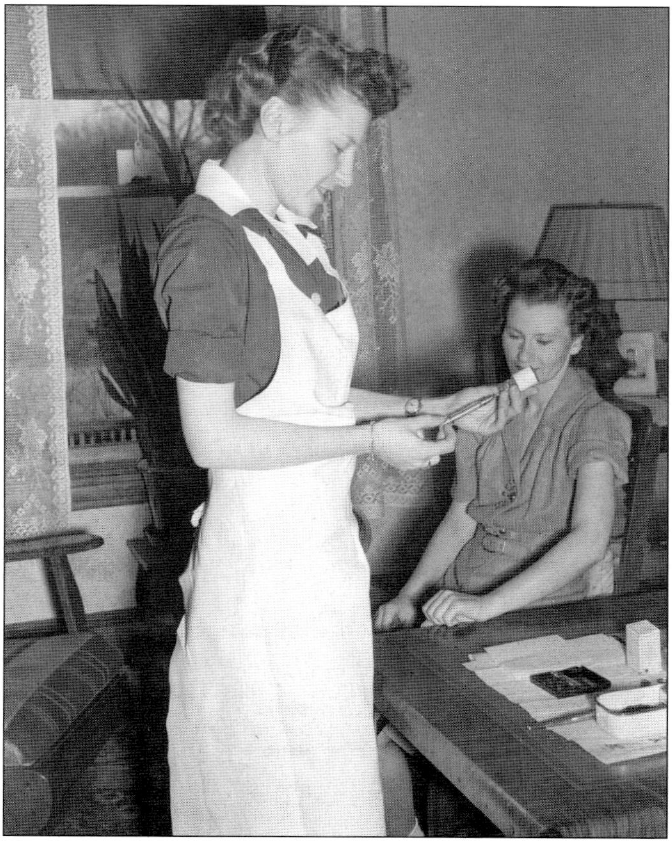

A visiting nurse prepares an injection for her patient in a private home. The nurses delivered what was known as "health in a bag." The VNA was founded by Anna Koch in 1910 and was a vital part of the health care community. Koch served as the director of the VNA for 25 years.

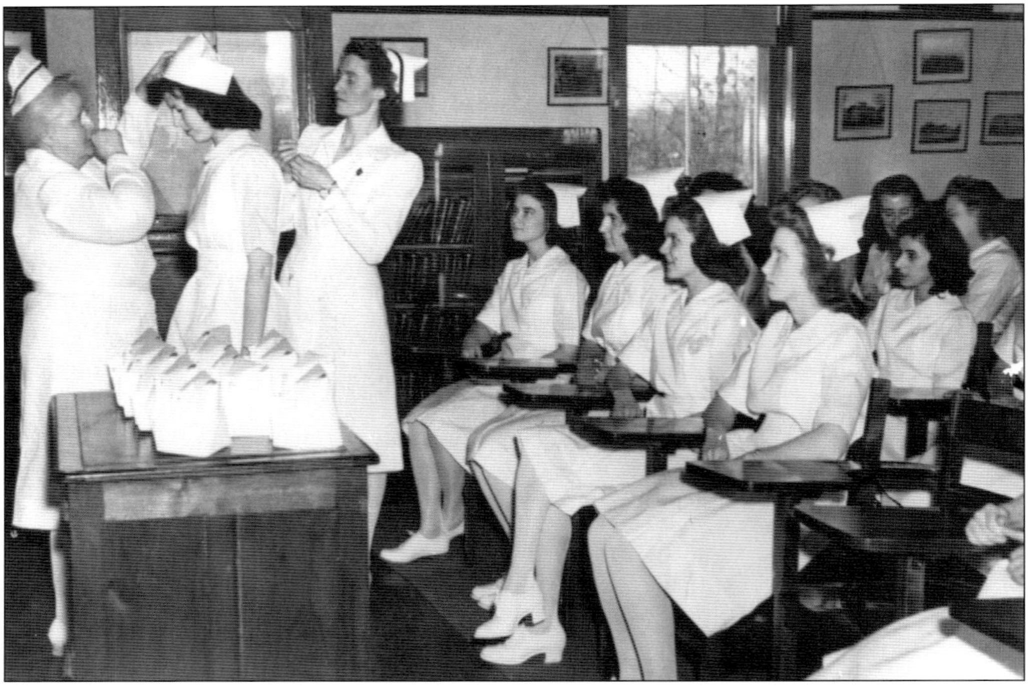

The FCPH School of Nursing held this capping ceremony in 1947. The formal ceremony occurred midway through a nursing student's freshman year and commemorates one of the most important milestones in a student's career. Student nurses wore plain white caps; one or two narrow black stripes indicated more seniority, and a single broad stripe on the cap marked a full-fledged graduate.

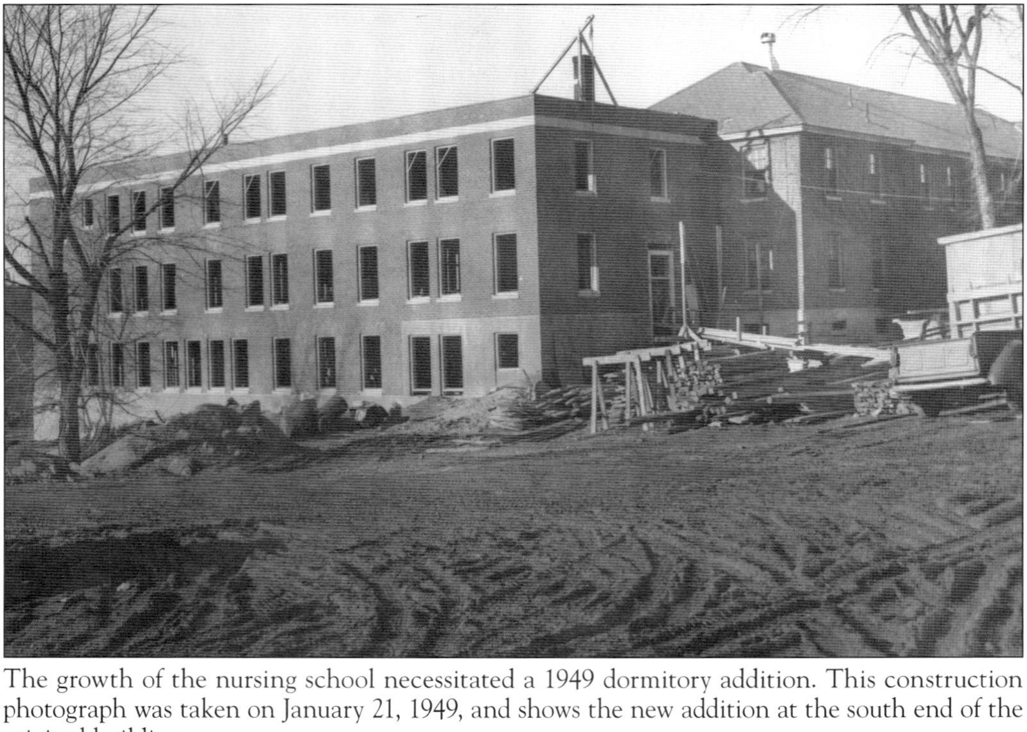

The growth of the nursing school necessitated a 1949 dormitory addition. This construction photograph was taken on January 21, 1949, and shows the new addition at the south end of the original building.

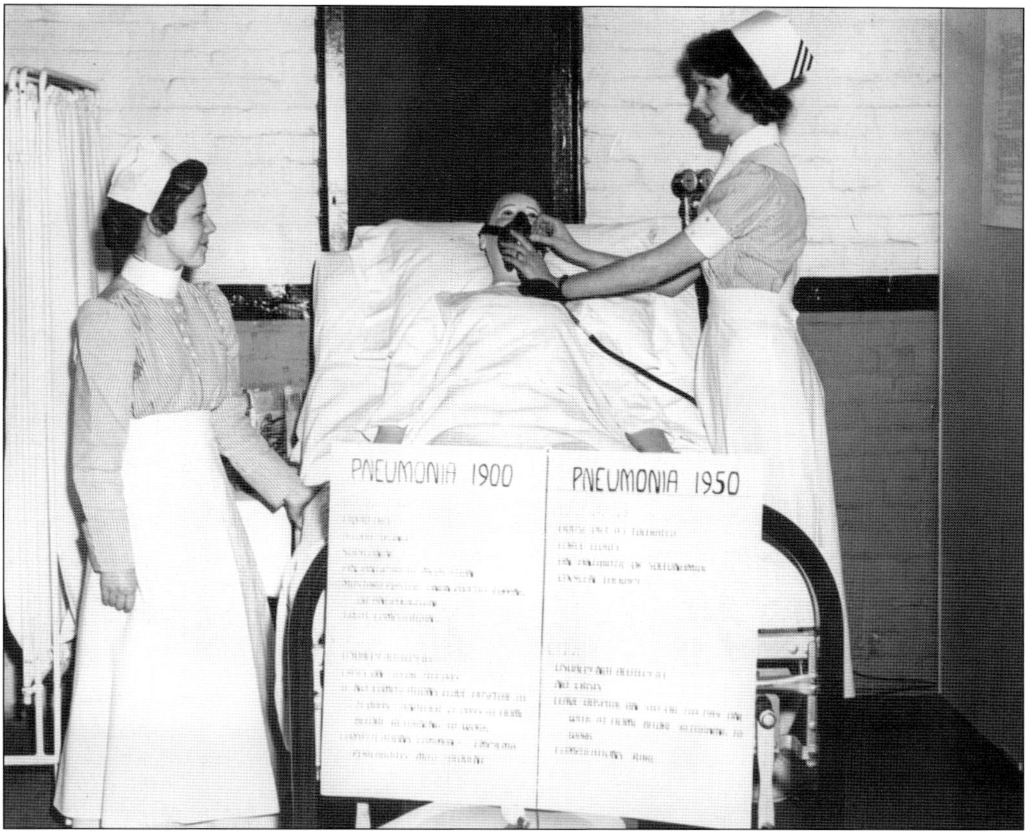

A nursing student watches a demonstration on how to provide care for a patient with pneumonia. Displayed in front of the patient's bed on a poster are the methods of care for pneumonia in 1900 and 1950, demonstrating the great advances in care. Pictured on the left is Marilyn A. Barry, class of 1953, and on the right is Helen Hannum O'Donnell, member of the class of 1951.

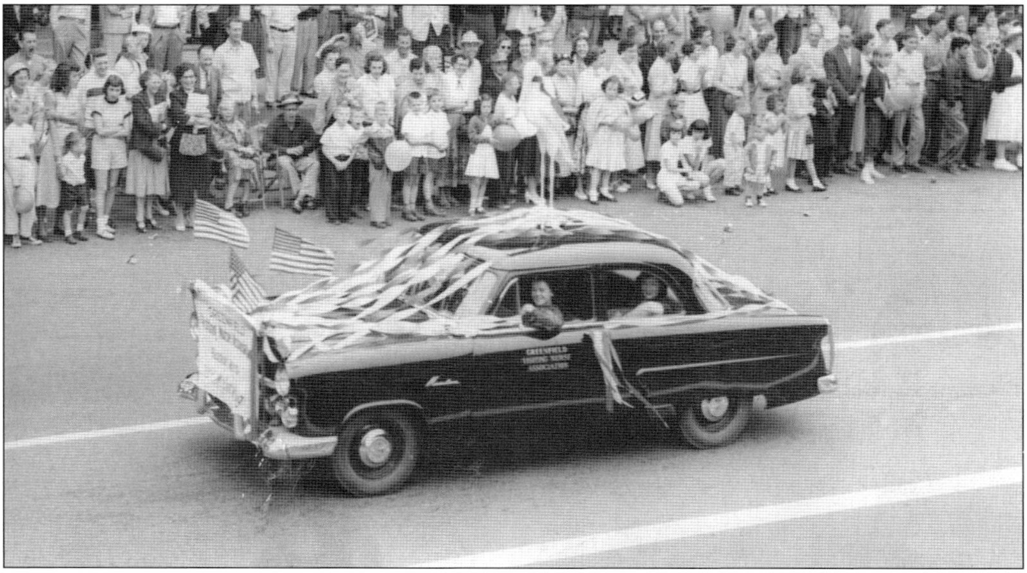

A Greenfield VNA vehicle is decked out for a parade through Greenfield in the mid-1950s.

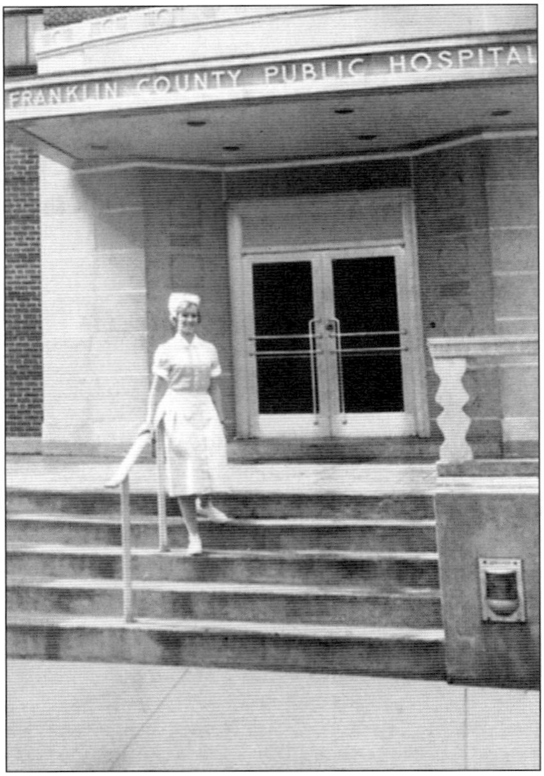

A hospital nurse stands at the front entrance of the Franklin County Public Hospital in the 1960s. This entrance to the hospital is still in use today, though it has been substantially remodeled throughout the years. In 1962, the school of nursing was accredited by the National League for Nursing, demonstrating that the program met all state and federal standards for nursing education and training.

This interior view of the living room in the nursing student building in 1960 shows student nurses discussing their studies with each other. The living room is simple in decoration but functional.

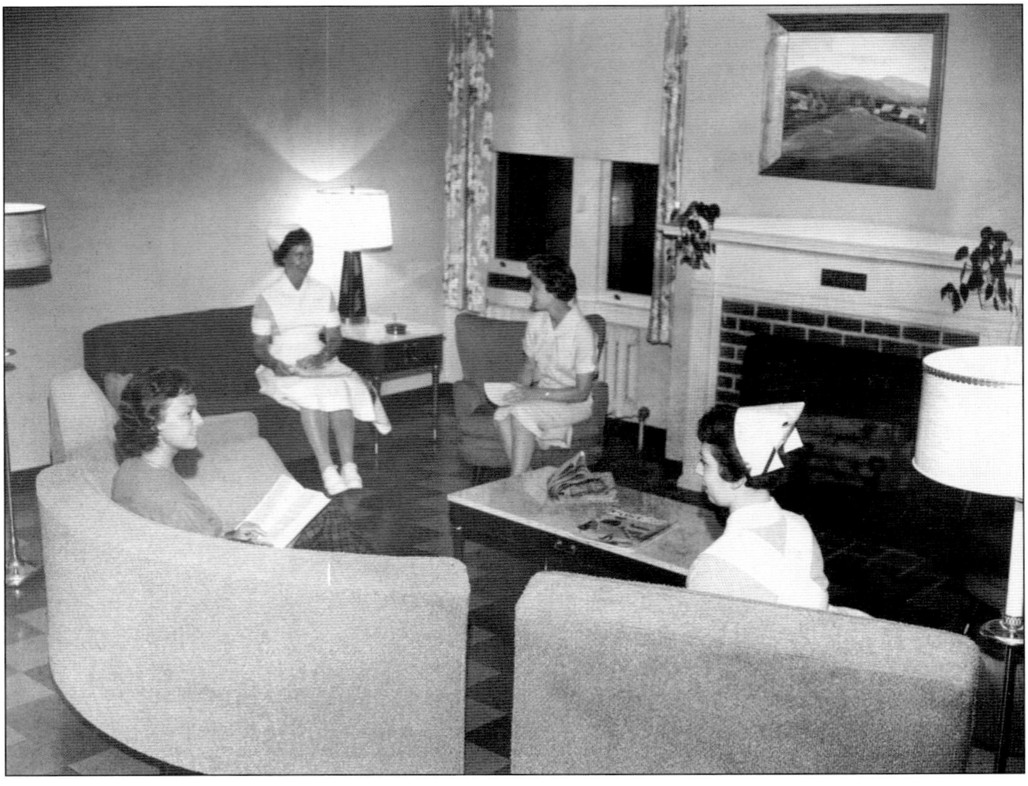

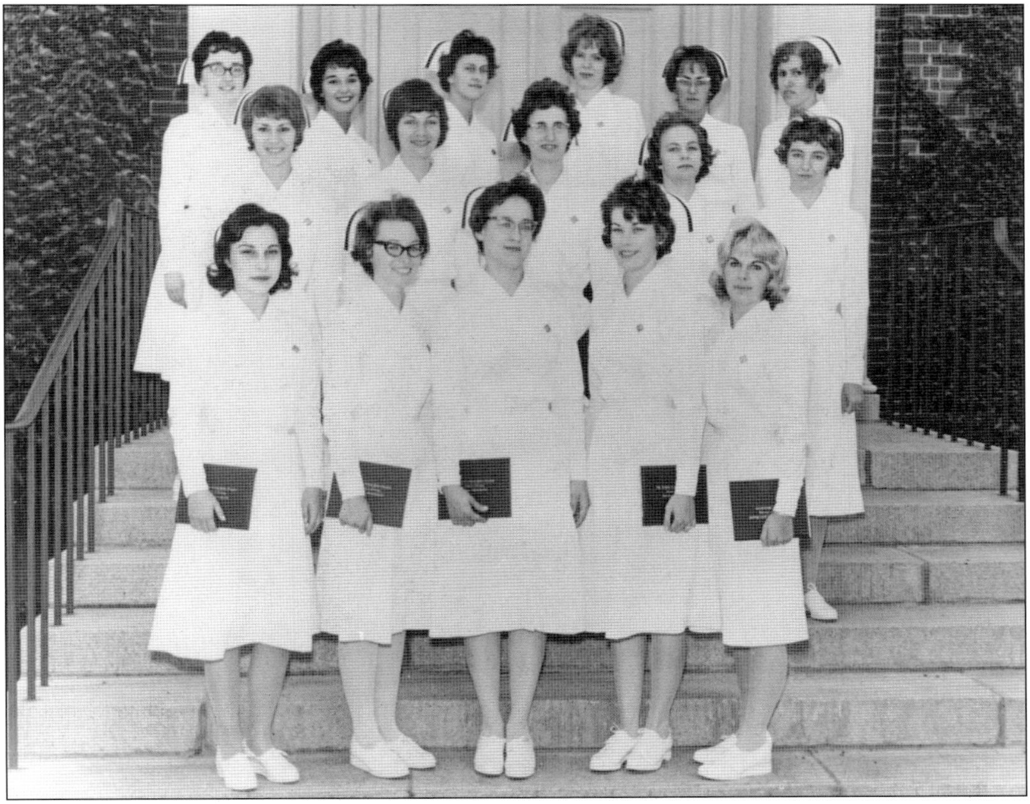

The FCPH School of Nursing class of 1963 is pictured on the steps of the hospital with their diplomas in hand. Note that the nursing cap on each nurse has the stripe of a graduate nurse. The Franklin County Public Hospital began training nurses in 1897 and ended with the class of 1965, with a total of 646 women graduating from the program. Greenfield Community College subsequently provided nursing education in Franklin County.

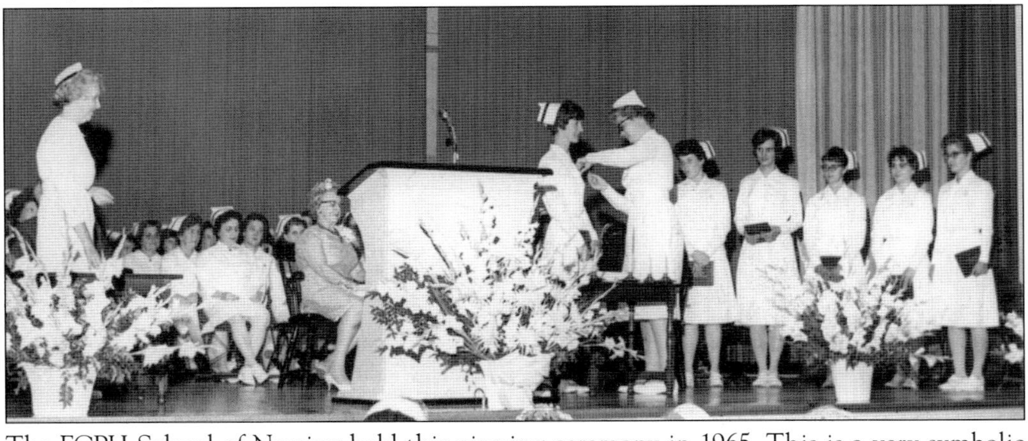

The FCPH School of Nursing held this pinning ceremony in 1965. This is a very symbolic ceremony held at or right before graduation from a nursing program and symbolizes the student entering the profession. Each nurse receives a pin from a faculty member of the program. The ceremony often included a prayer, greetings from the board of trustees and professional staff, a formal address from the director of nursing, recitation of the Nightingale Pledge, and a reception hosted by the Board of Organized Work.

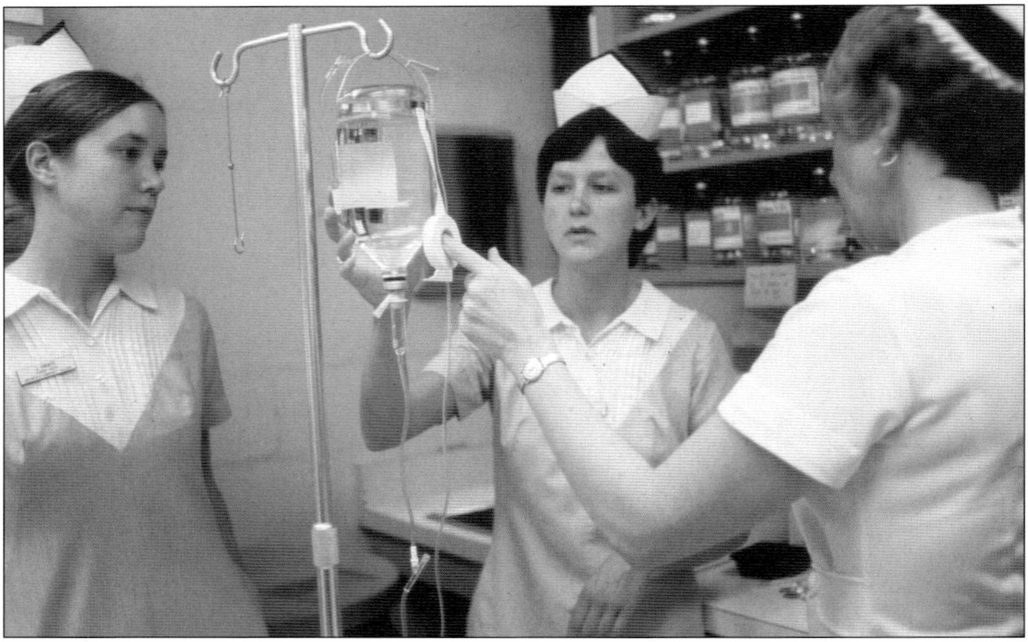

Nursing students are preparing an intravenous medication contained in a glass bottle. To prepare the medication, a nurse needed to calculate the drops per minute for the medication and adjust the roller clamp on the tubing accordingly. The white tape on the bottle being held by the nurse was used to mark off times when a certain amount of medication was due to have been administered. These processes were used before today's technology of highly specialized, programmable pumps.

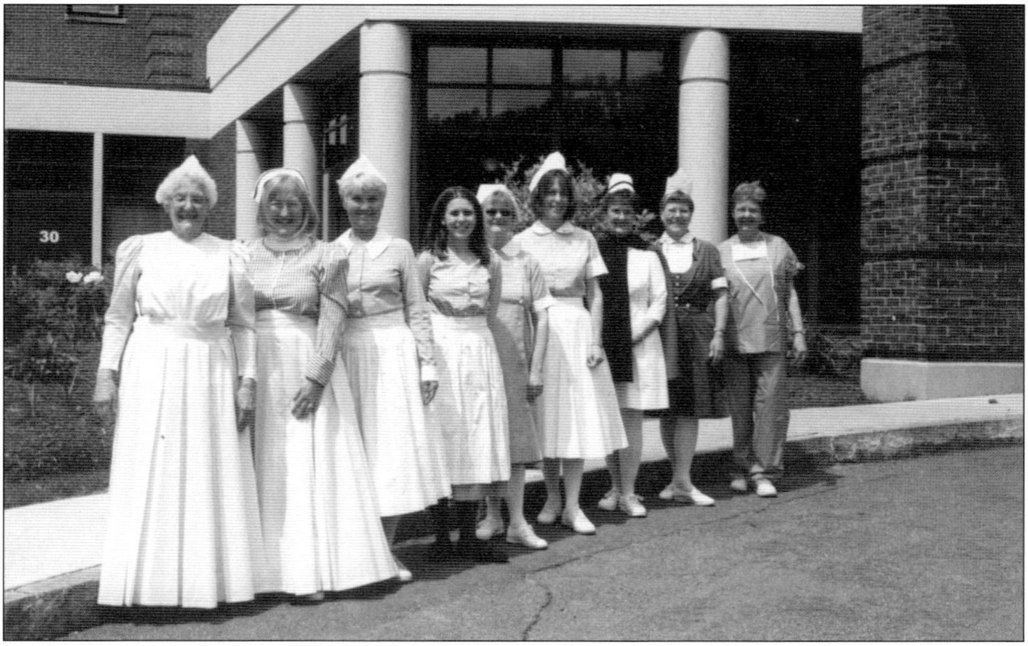

Baystate Franklin Medical Center staff wear nursing uniforms from throughout the years to celebrate Nurses' Week. The nursing uniform collection is owned by Deborah Wheeler (second from left), a staff member at Baystate Franklin Medical Center. Wheeler has graciously shared her collection several times with the hospital for different celebrations of nursing.

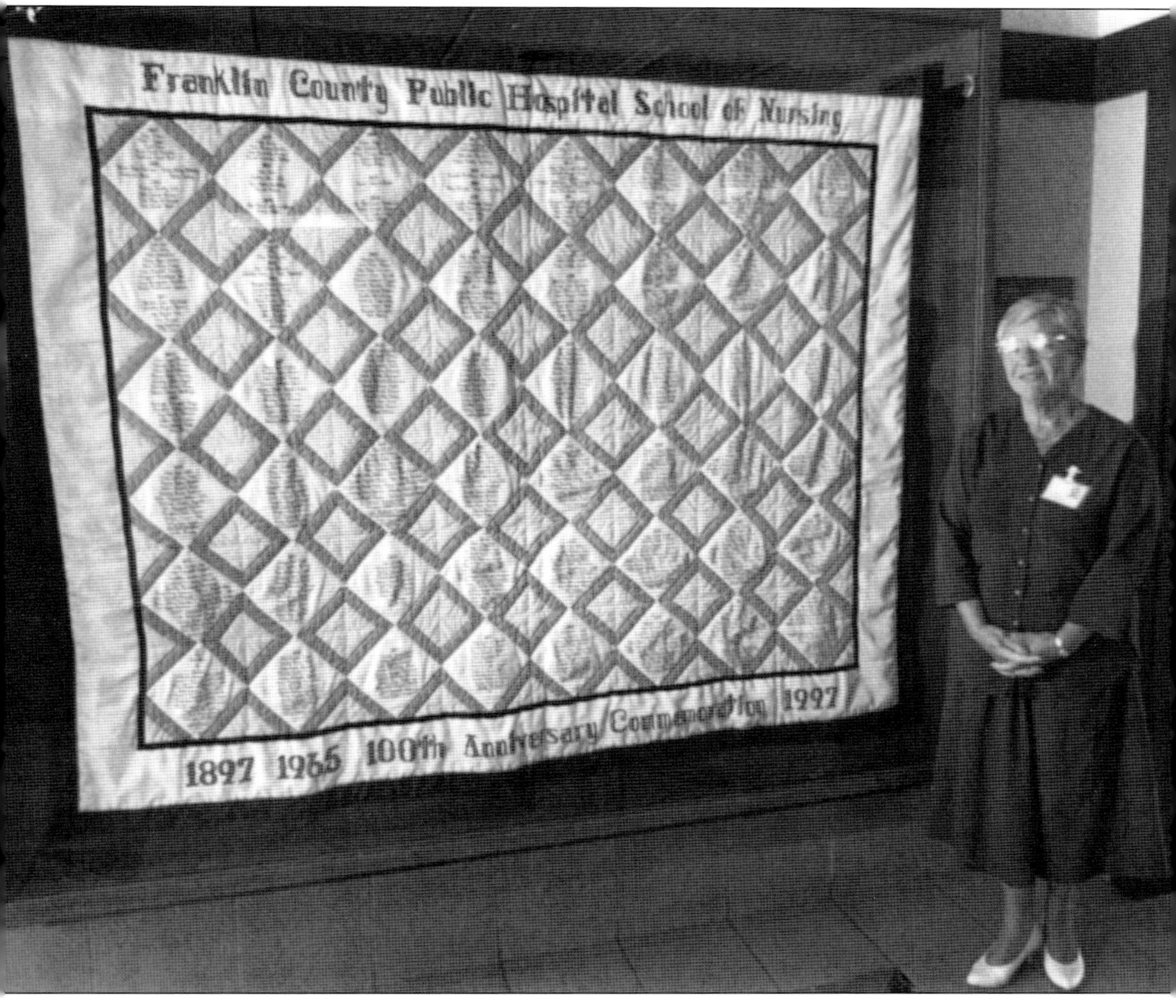

Esther Purinton of Charlemont (FCPH School of Nursing class of 1956) stands in front of the quilt bearing the names of the graduates of the school. Purinton worked for the hospital for over 33 years and was an active member of the School of Nursing Alumni Society. The quilt hangs today outside the hospital's main conference rooms off the main lobby. It was given to the hospital in 1997 to commemorate the 100th anniversary of the school of nursing.

School of Nursing

Director

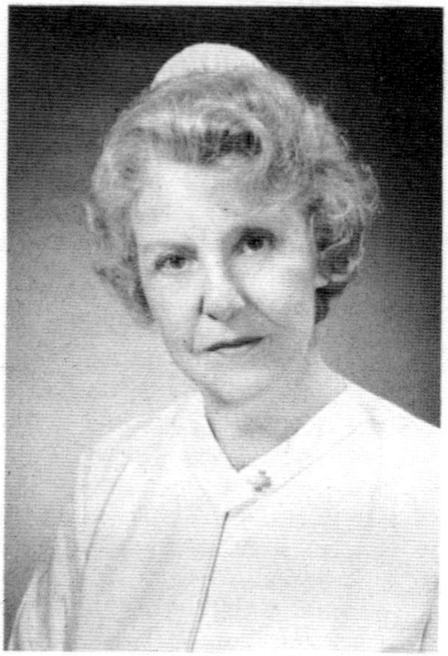

Ellen G. Creamer
1956 to Present

Faculty

Associate Director

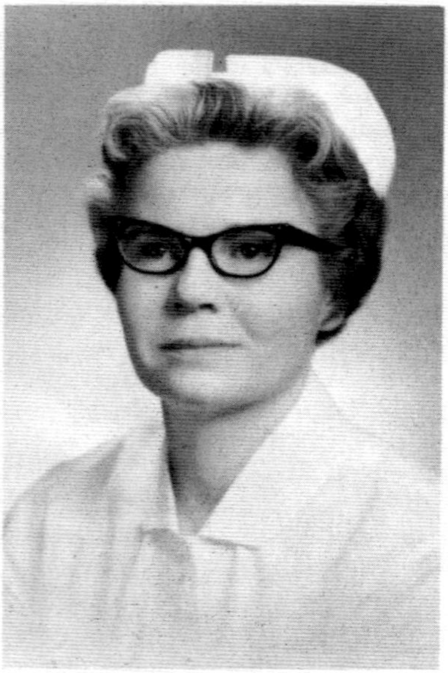

Marjorie Heywood
1957 to Present

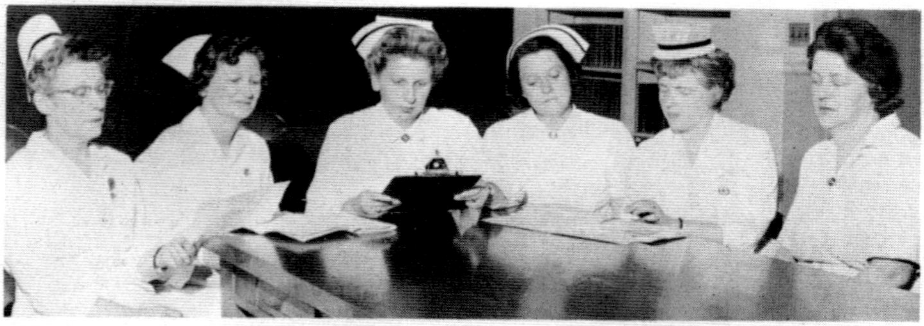

Regina H. Babineau, Dorothy N. Saulnier, Dorothy J. Telega, Louise M. Sessler, Peggy D. Muscente, Elizabeth B. Damon.

Faculty of the FCPH School of Nursing in the early 1960s included director Ellen G. Creamer (top right), Marjorie Heywood (top left), and, from left to right, Regina H. Babineau, Dorothy N. Salvinier, Dorothy J. Telega, Louise M. Sessler, Peggy D. Muscente, and Elizabeth B. Damon.

Five

The Board of Organized Work

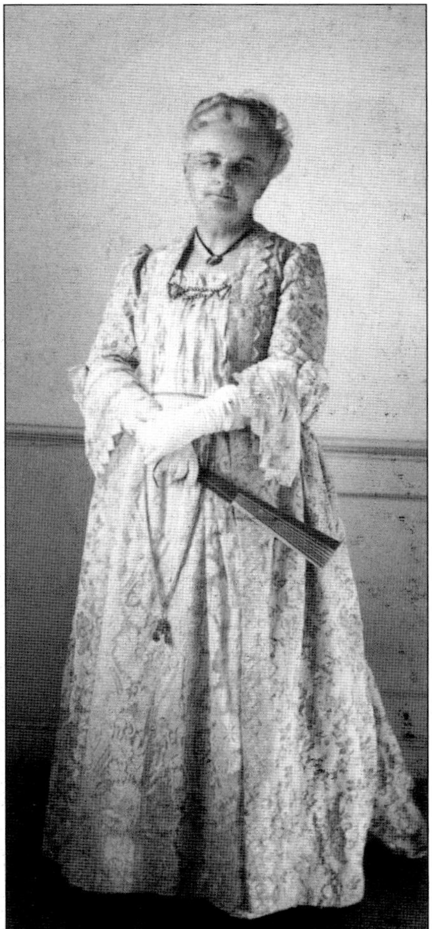

Charlotte Alice Baker (1833–1909), an educator and historian, was an early supporter of FCPH and was involved in many fundraising events. Her home in Deerfield, known as the Frary House, was used for many of these functions. (HD.)

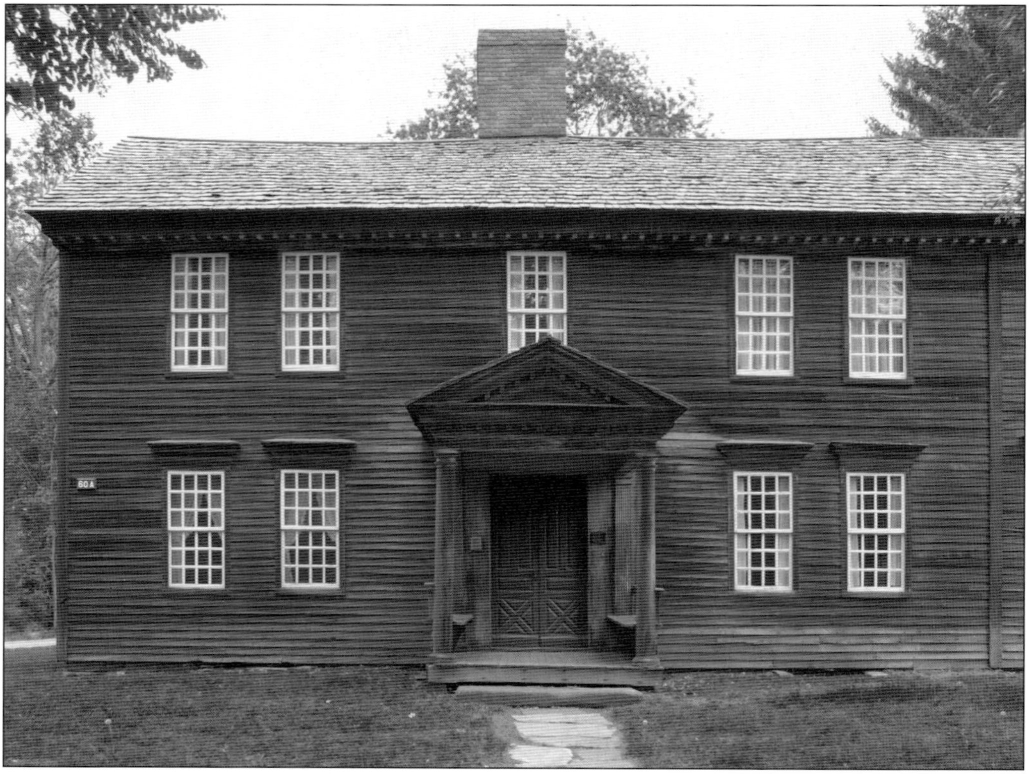

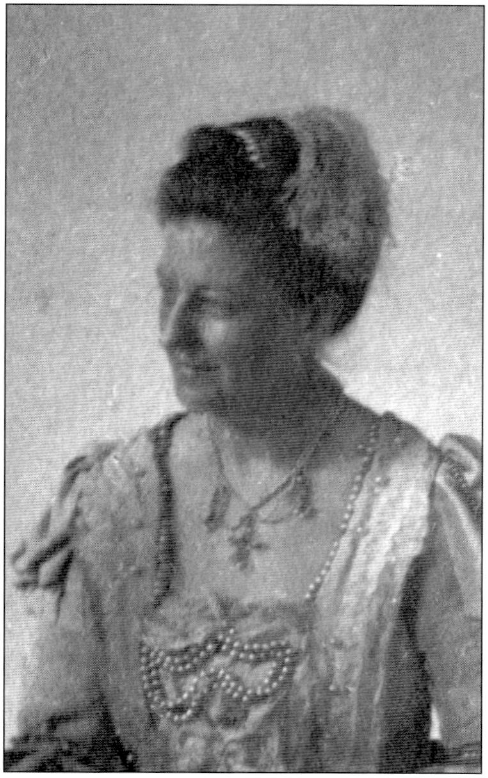

The Frary House, owned by C. Alice Baker, was built around 1750 and restored in 1892 as a way of demonstrating the Arts and Crafts movement in Deerfield. This was the site of many fundraisers held on behalf of FCPH. One of the most unusual events took place in October 1908. Known as the Bizarre Bazar, it raised over $800 for the hospital building fund. More than 400 people joined in this event, which included a vaudeville performance, several musical performances, a farmer's market, a silhouette artist, a luncheon, and an evening dance held at the town hall. (HD.)

Emma Lewis Coleman (1853–1942) was the organizer of the Bizarre Bazar, held at the Frary House in 1908. Based on the success of this fundraiser, Coleman, a resident of both Boston and Deerfield, continued to hold various events to aid in the hospital building fund. She was also a well-known photographer and author and a serious researcher. She resided with C. Alice Baker while living in Deerfield; the two gathered information about the Deerfield children taken captive in February 1704 by making several journeys to Canada. (HD.)

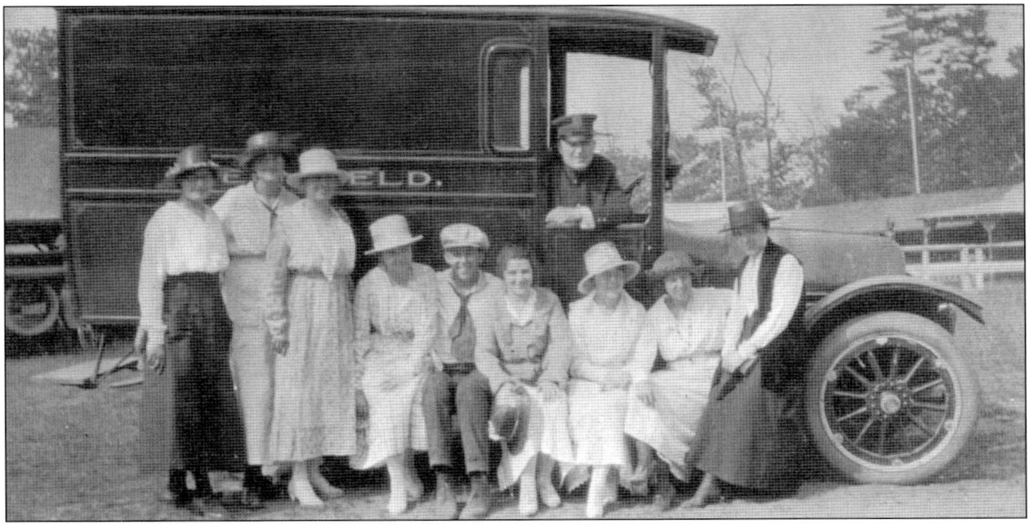

Prior to FCPH having its own ambulance, the Greenfield Police patrol wagon was used to transport patients to the hospital. Pictured here in the 1920s are several townspeople along with a police officer.

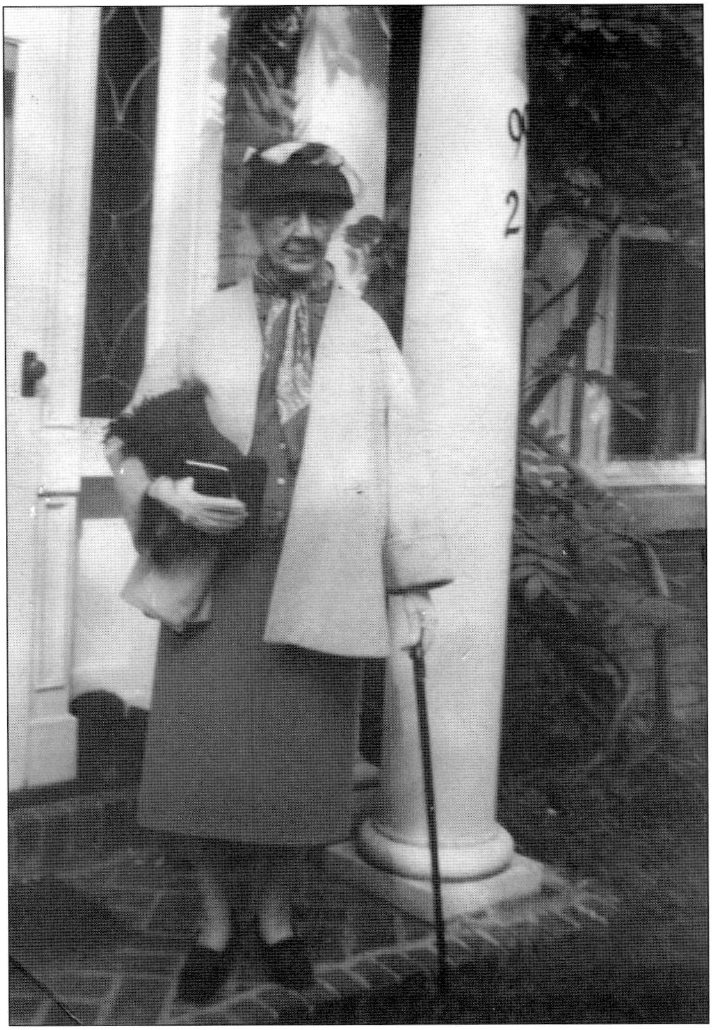

Pictured is Alice Newton Judd (1870–1973), who established a fund in 1925 for the first motorized ambulance for FCPH. The board raised $1,390 toward the purchase of this ambulance. In later years, the Judd Fund was diverted to other uses when it became too costly for the board to maintain the ambulance for the hospital. (Courtesy of Doug Lyman.)

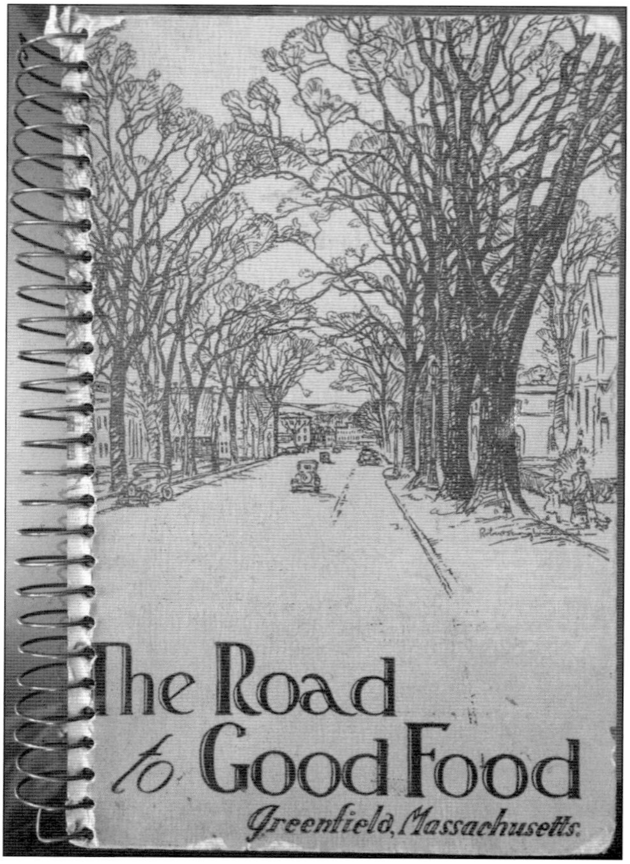

This cookbook was published in June 1935 by the Board of Organized Work (BOOW) as one of its fundraisers. The book was in honor of the hospital's 40th anniversary and included all handwritten recipes. It was also illustrated by artists of the community. Due to its popularity, subsequent editions were published in November 1935, November 1936, and July 1946. Two additional cookbooks were also published by the BOOW in later years.

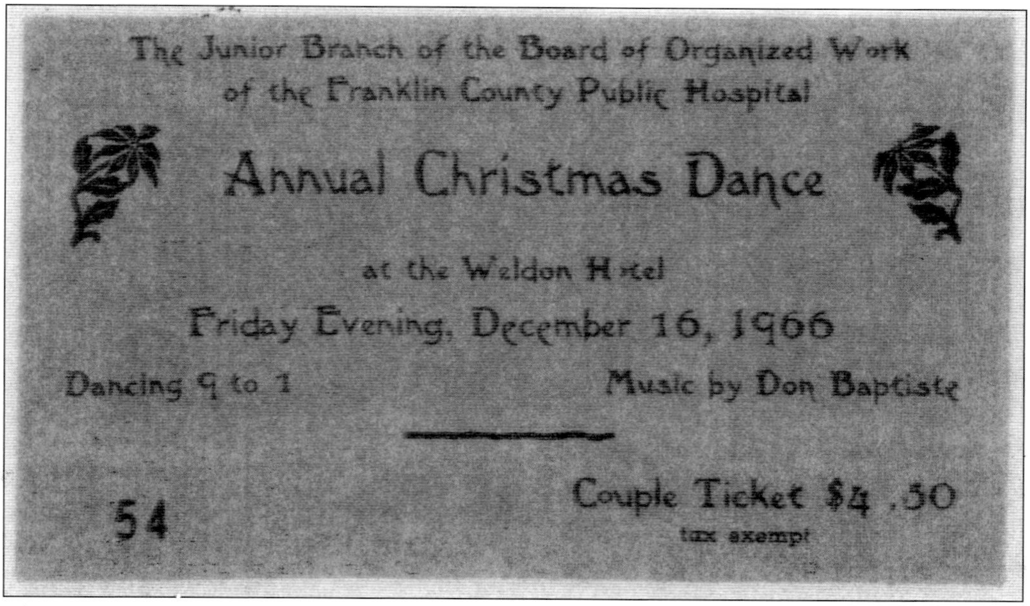

The BOOW held many dances over the years as a popular way to raise money for the hospital. In 1966, the Junior Branch held its annual Christmas dance at the Weldon Hotel. This "couple ticket" cost $4.50.

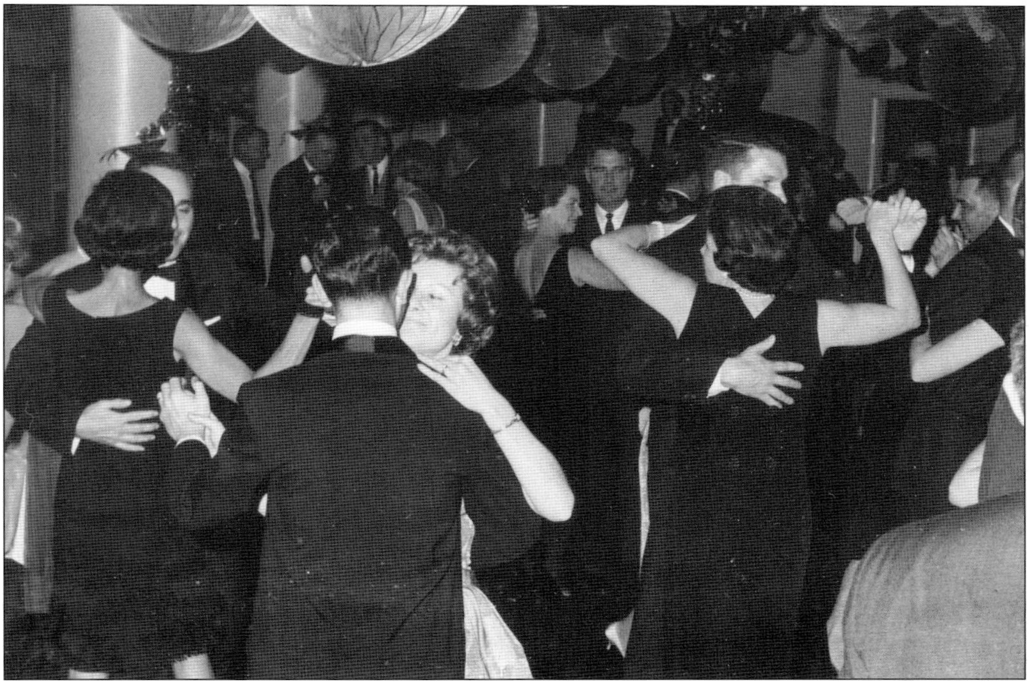

Pictured is one of the dances organized by the BOOW as a fundraising event around 1965. This popular event was held for many years at the Weldon Hotel, and many of the town's business leaders, physicians, and lawyers attended in support of FCPH.

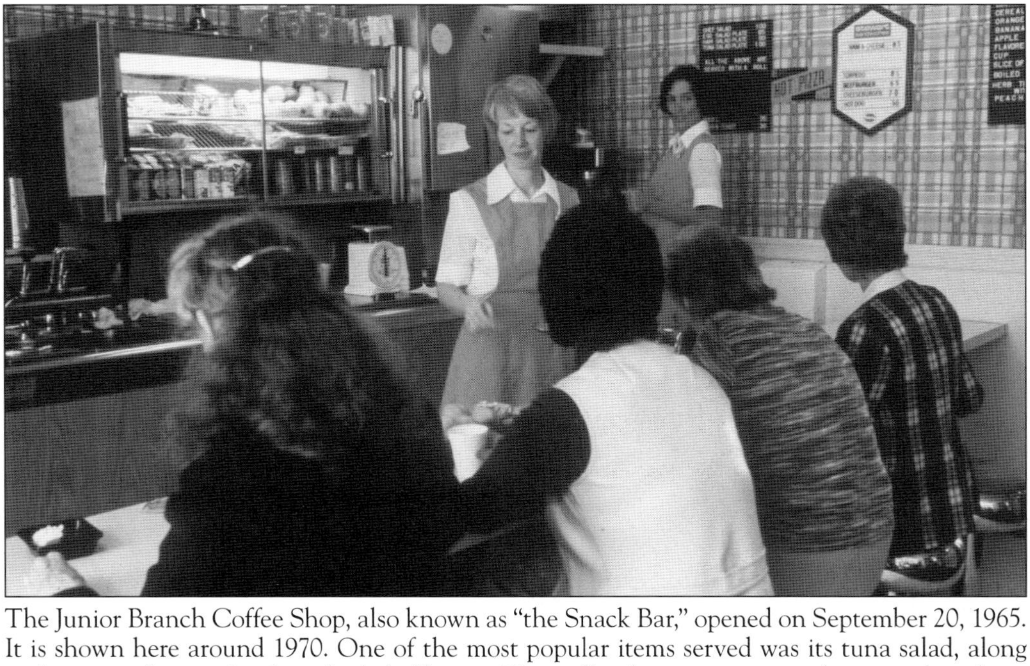

The Junior Branch Coffee Shop, also known as "the Snack Bar," opened on September 20, 1965. It is shown here around 1970. One of the most popular items served was its tuna salad, along with many other sandwich and salad offerings. The coffee shop was open six days a week and was run entirely by volunteers except for a few weeks in the summer when a paid worker was hired. In July 1966, after less than one year of the coffee shop's existence, the Junior Branch was able to donate $1,500 to the hospital.

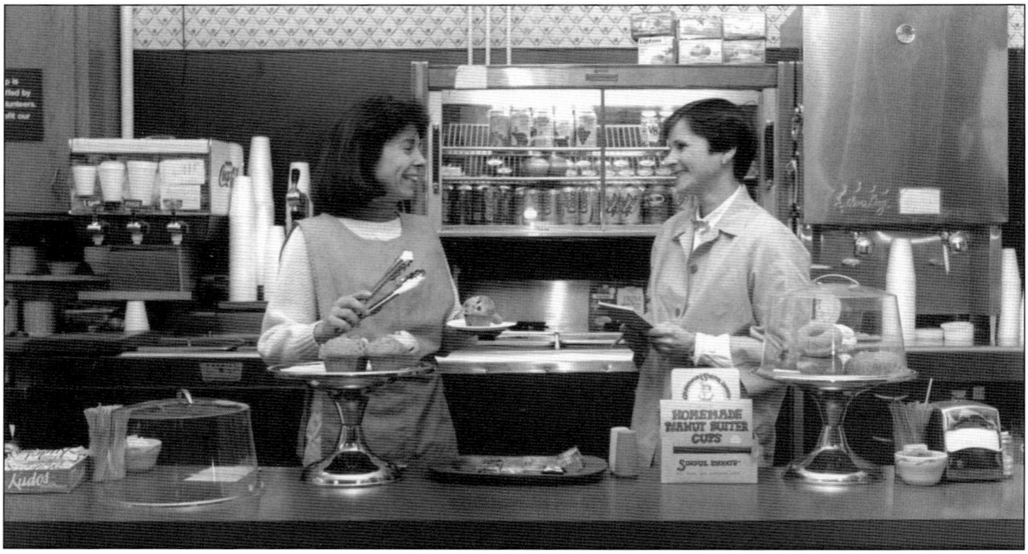

Barbara Killeen and Cherry Goodwin, Junior Branch volunteers pictured here in the early 1990s, work the counter at the coffee shop in one of the last years it was open. The intent of the Junior Branch, which was begun in 1918, was to engage women under 40 in volunteerism with a focus on fundraising for pediatric patients.

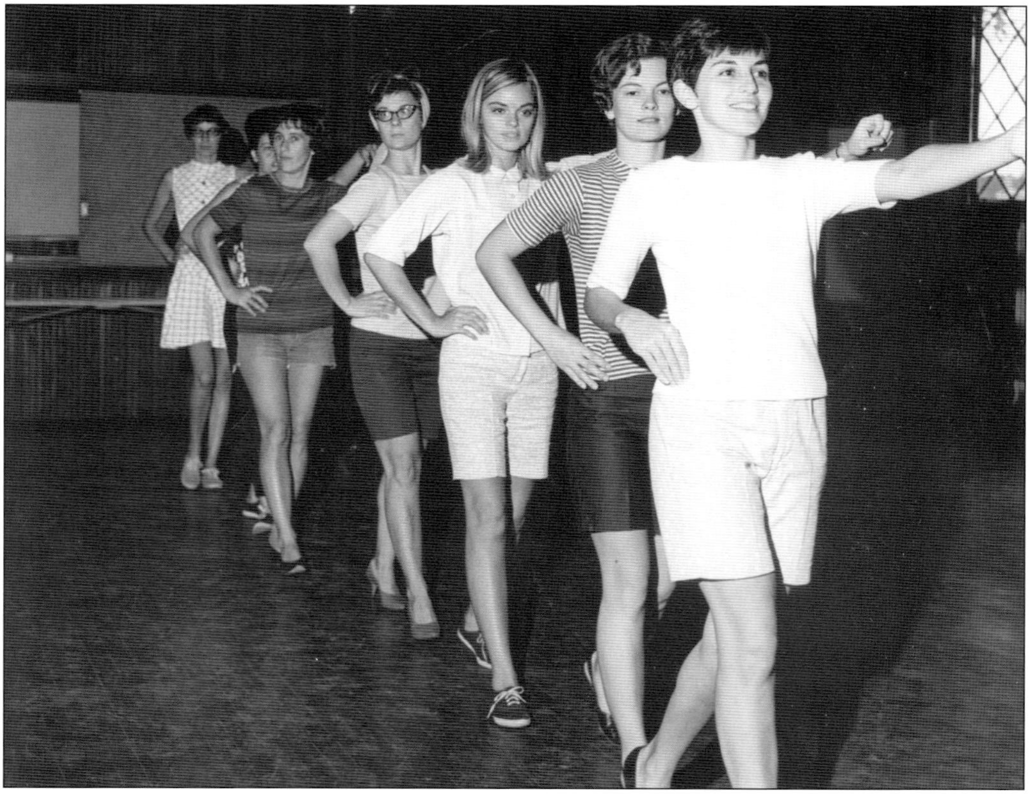

The Junior Branch was also responsible for The Follies, another popular fundraising event for the hospital. This picture from 1968, with the line led by former member Dorothy Fitch, shows the group practicing a dance routine.

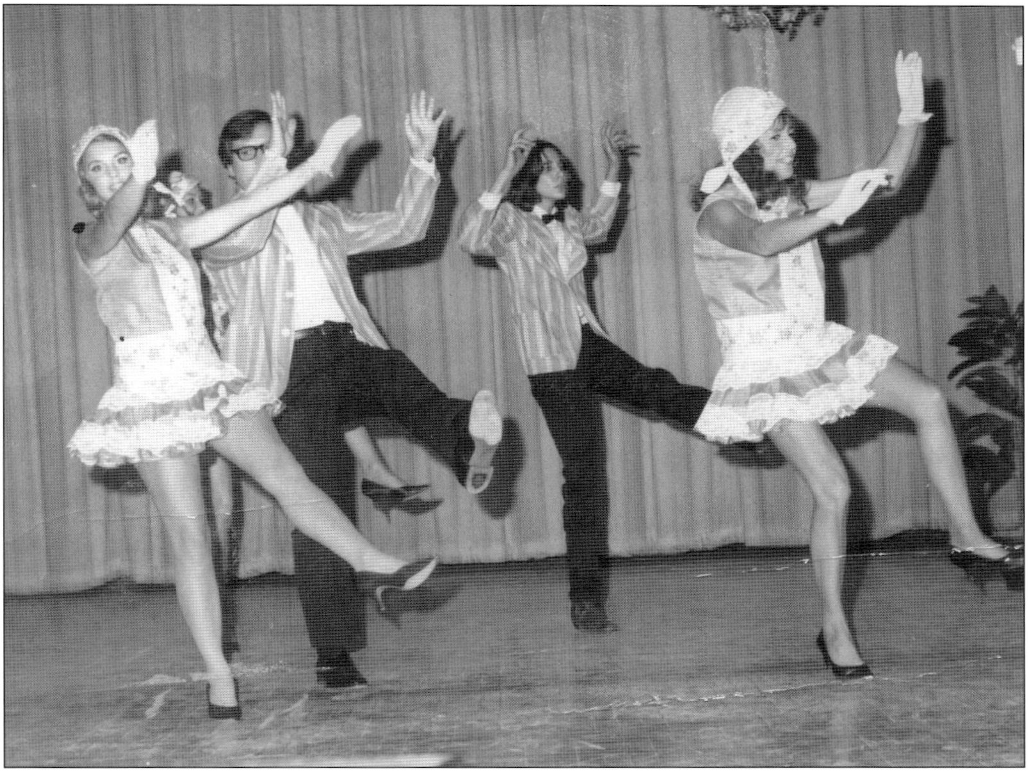

Here is another picture from a practice session for the 1968 Follies, which included many of the Junior Branch members. These fun-filled events were held many times over the years and proved to be very successful fundraisers for the Junior Branch. Money raised purchased such items as x-ray equipment and monitors for the ICU and kidney dialysis units, and also allowed for expanded space for the laboratory along with funds for the new surgery building in 1972.

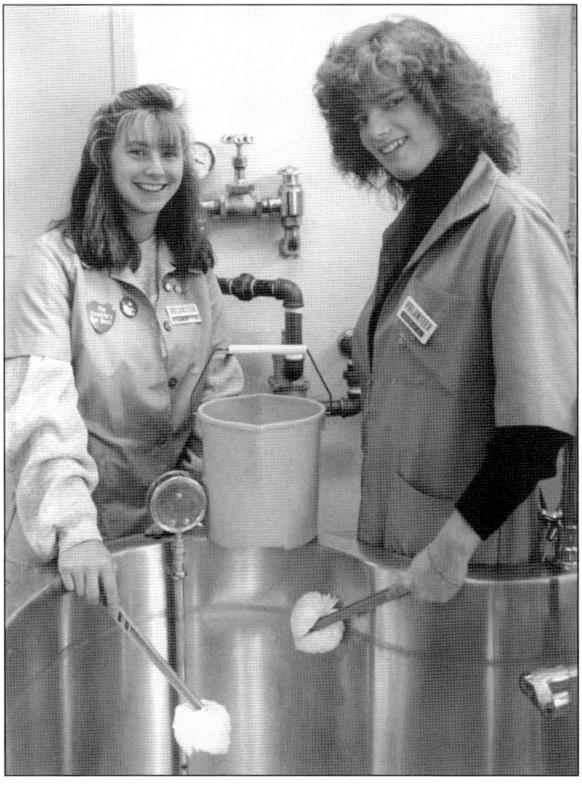

The student volunteers (formerly known as candy stripers) pictured in this 1980s photograph are Bonnie Drown (left) and Angela Earl. They were given the task of cleaning the hydrotherapy tub, which was used in the Rehabilitation Department.

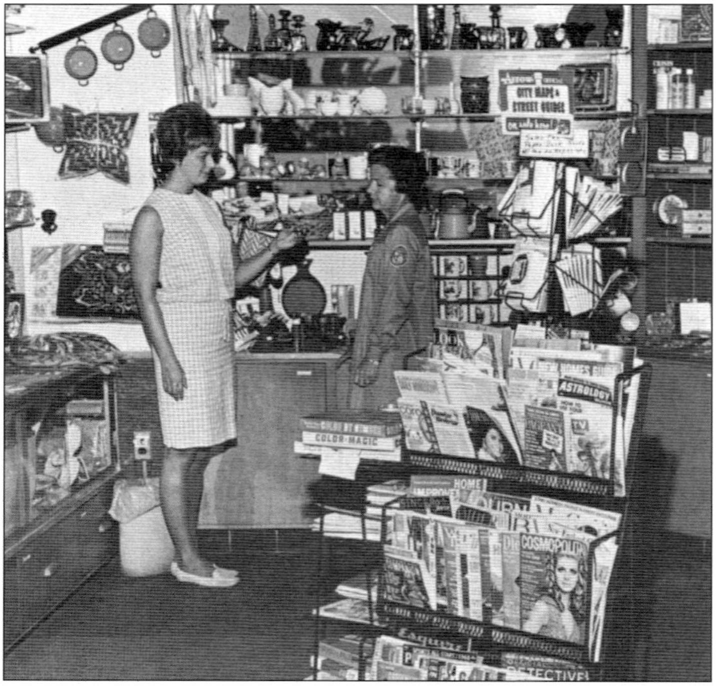

The mainstay of BOOW efforts has been the gift shop, located in the main lobby. In this c. 1980 photograph, a customer talks with a volunteer. A variety of gifts and periodicals are available for purchase.

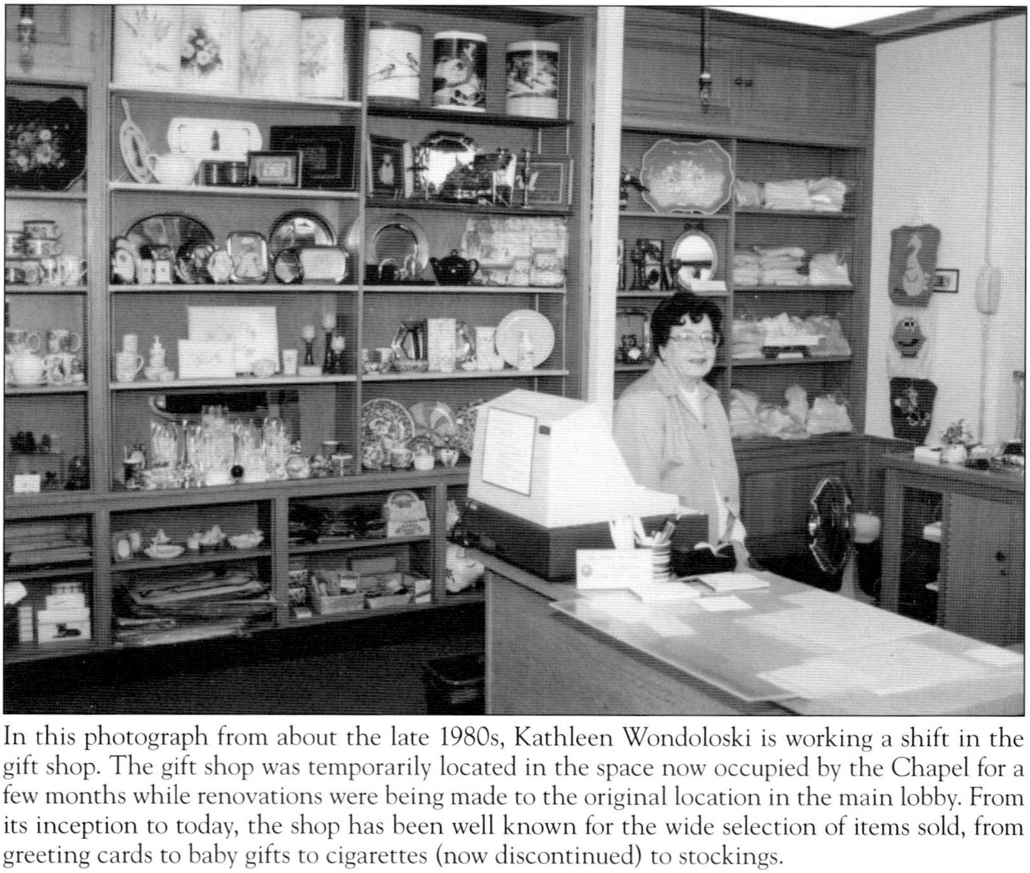

In this photograph from about the late 1980s, Kathleen Wondoloski is working a shift in the gift shop. The gift shop was temporarily located in the space now occupied by the Chapel for a few months while renovations were being made to the original location in the main lobby. From its inception to today, the shop has been well known for the wide selection of items sold, from greeting cards to baby gifts to cigarettes (now discontinued) to stockings.

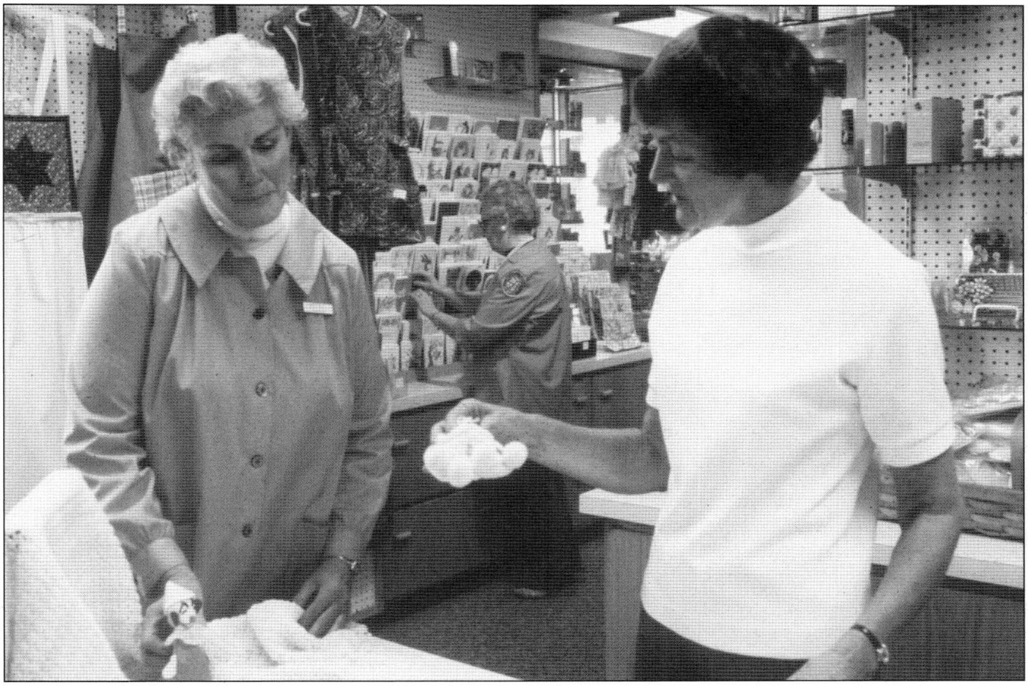

Members of the BOOW, now known as the Baystate Franklin Auxiliary (BFA), are identified by their pink jackets. They are the volunteers who work in the gift shop and also in the surgery reception area greeting patients and family members. Pictured here are two volunteers in the gift shop. Aprons displayed were locally made by members of the BOOW, and this tradition continues today.

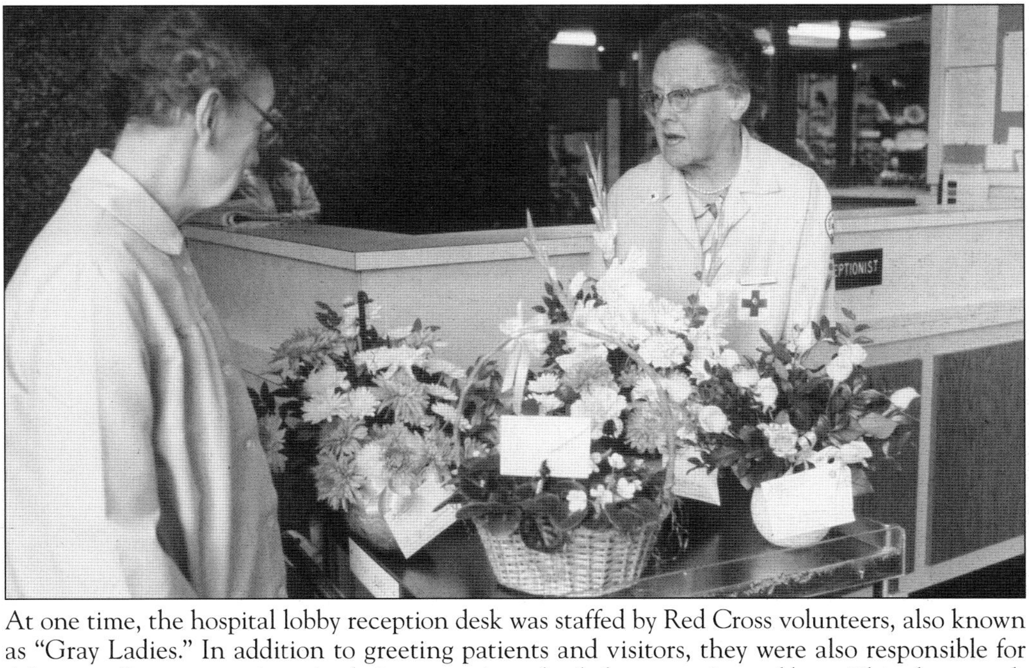

At one time, the hospital lobby reception desk was staffed by Red Cross volunteers, also known as "Gray Ladies." In addition to greeting patients and visitors, they were also responsible for delivering flowers to patients in their rooms via a wheeled cart, as pictured here. This photograph was taken prior to the lobby renovations made in the early 1990s.

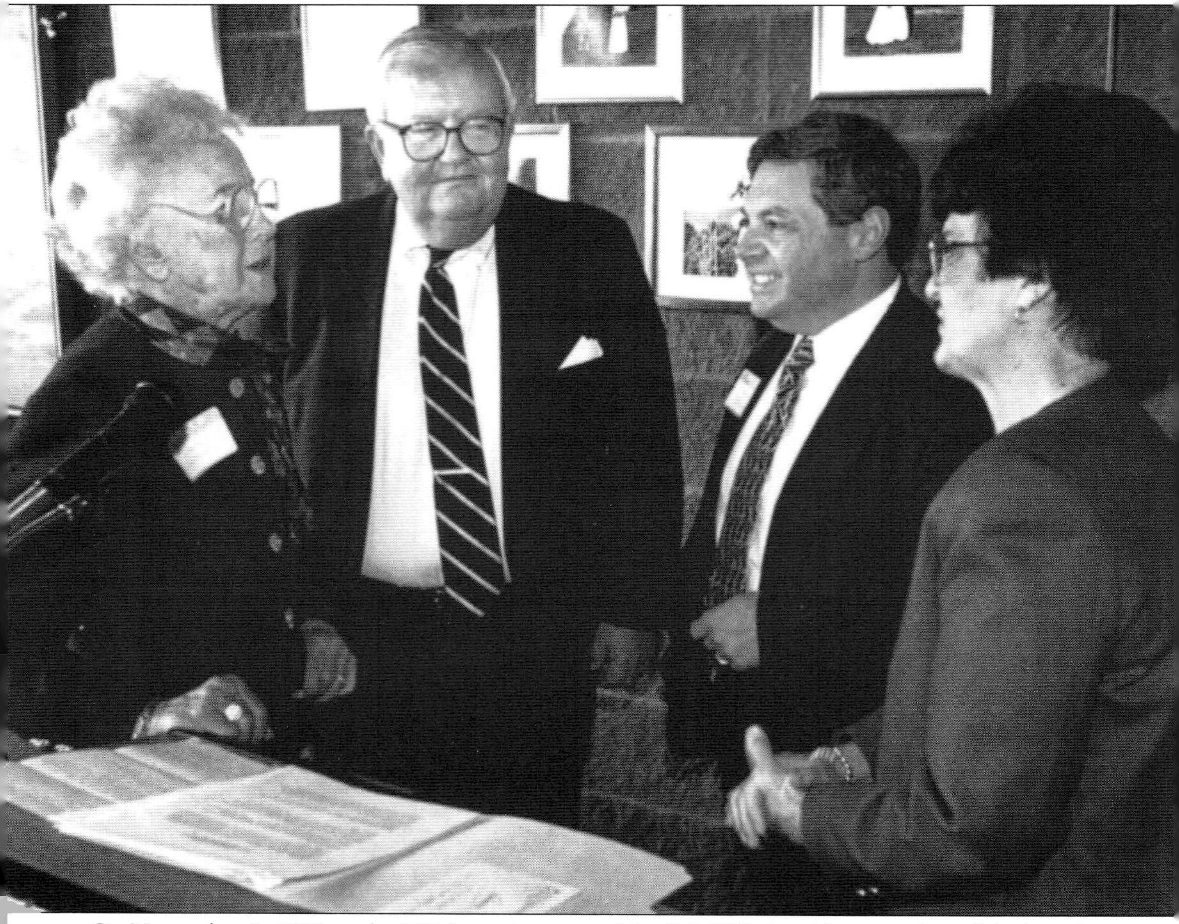

On November 6, 1995, at the 100th anniversary of the BOOW, the oldest member of the board at that time, Dorothy Affhauser (far left), is getting ready to present a check for $100,000 to David Currey, chairman of the board of directors, and Harlan Smith, hospital president. At far right is Elaine Chichester, a BOOW/BFA member since 1983 and president from 1994 to 1995. She continues to be a very active volunteer at BFMC. (GR.)

Six

The Postwar Years

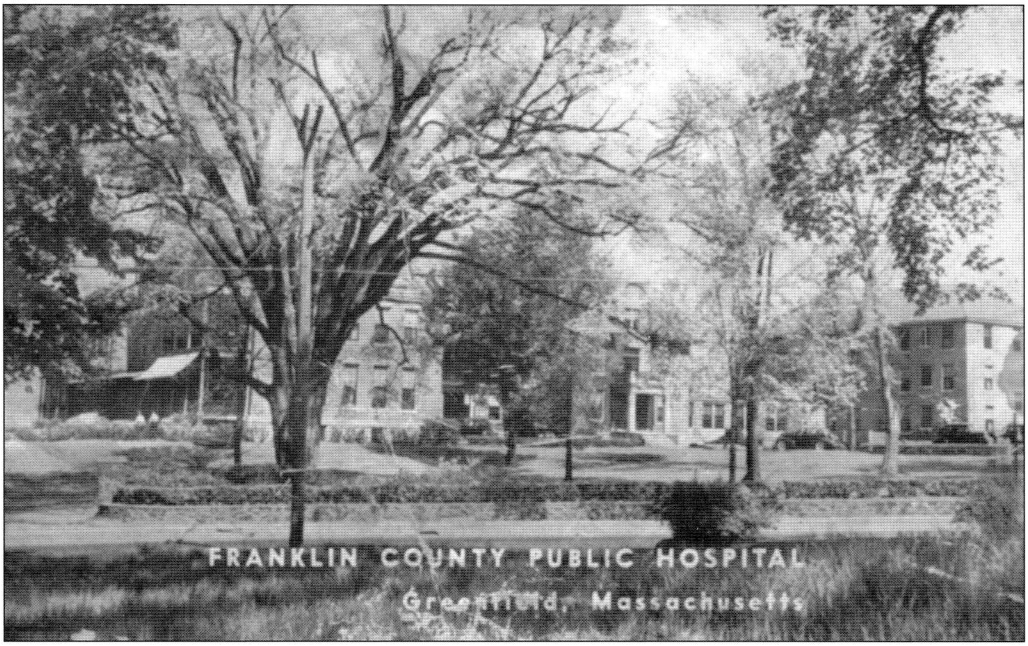

This fundraising card, issued in February 1946, shows the South, Administration, and North Wings of the hospital as viewed from across High Street (Massachusetts Route 2), then the main road between Boston and Albany, New York. The back of the card describes the increase in the number of patients served and notes that more than $8,100 per year is spent to care for patients outside Greenfield itself. The fundraising message is based on the concept that "responsibility for care of these patients logically belongs to those communities."

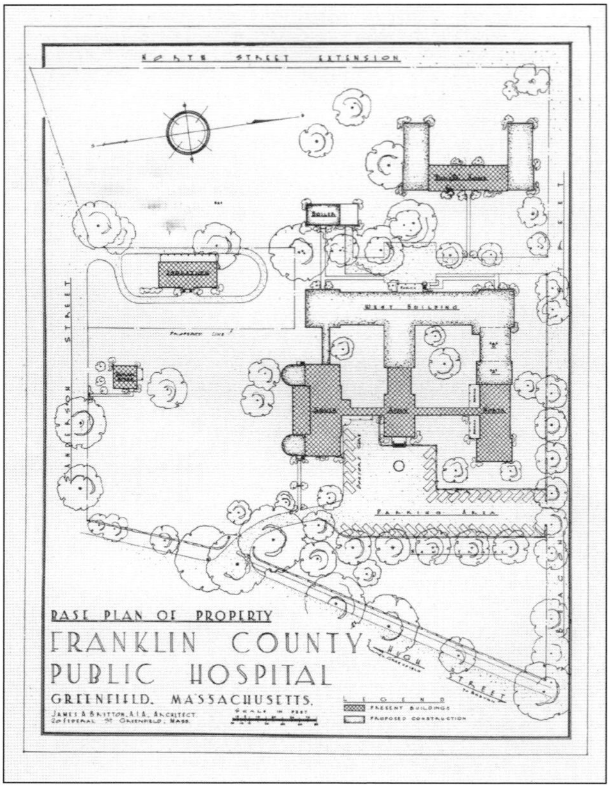

This is an early plan for hospital expansion drawn up by local architect James A. Britton. The crosshatched portions represent existing buildings. This expansion plan envisioned a new West Building connecting to the three existing structures, along with expansion of the steam plant and the nursing school. Ultimately, a different approach was taken.

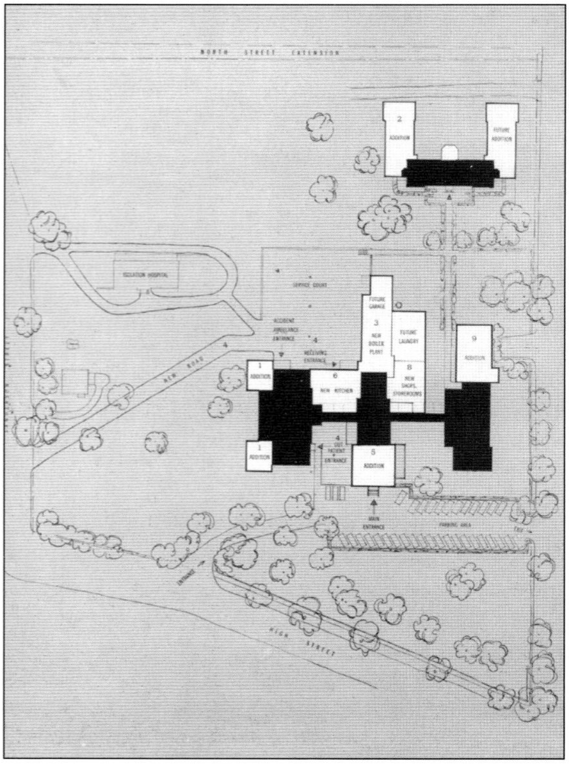

By 1945, the Health, Hope, and Happiness campaign had kicked off, and plans had changed markedly. The sun porches on the South Wing were to be enlarged and enclosed (1), new wings were proposed for the nursing school (2), the North Wing was expanded (9), and a cluster of new facilities (3 through 8) surrounded the 1910-vintage Administration Building. While closer to what was eventually constructed, this plan was never fully executed aside from the dormitory added to the south side of the nursing school in 1949.

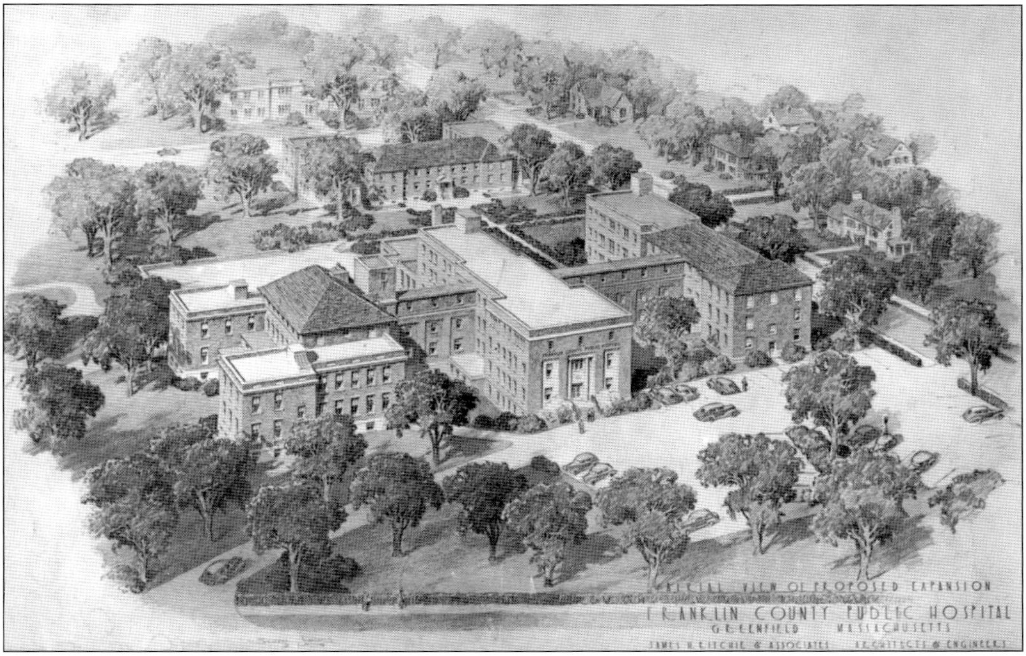

This architect's rendering gives a bird's-eye view of the 1945 plan. The expanded South Building would accommodate a new children's ward, a modernized Obstetric Department, and a new "accident ward." The Central Building would feature modern operating rooms, a new medical library, conference and staff rooms, a new kitchen, and a new boiler plant. The North Building would expand by 29 beds.

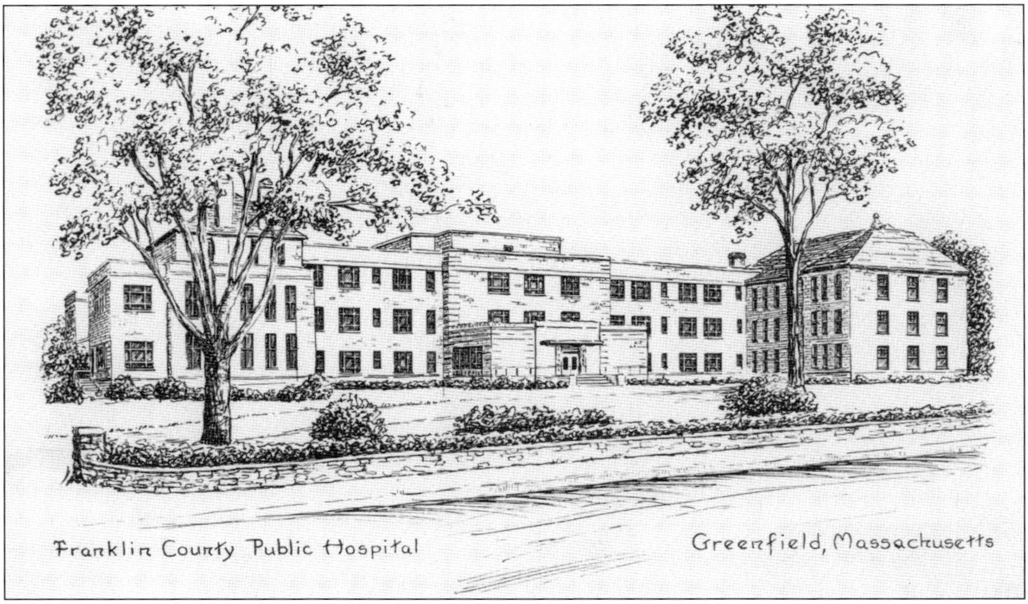

The fundraising campaign was structured to encourage 10 quarterly payments beginning in the last quarter of 1946 and ending in 1949. The brochure stated that this was "NOT an annual campaign" but a one-time appeal. Donors were advised that the quarterly payment plan covered tax deductions over four years, budgeted giving, and permitted a larger investment. This architect's rendering, from later in the fundraising campaign, accurately depicts what was finally built.

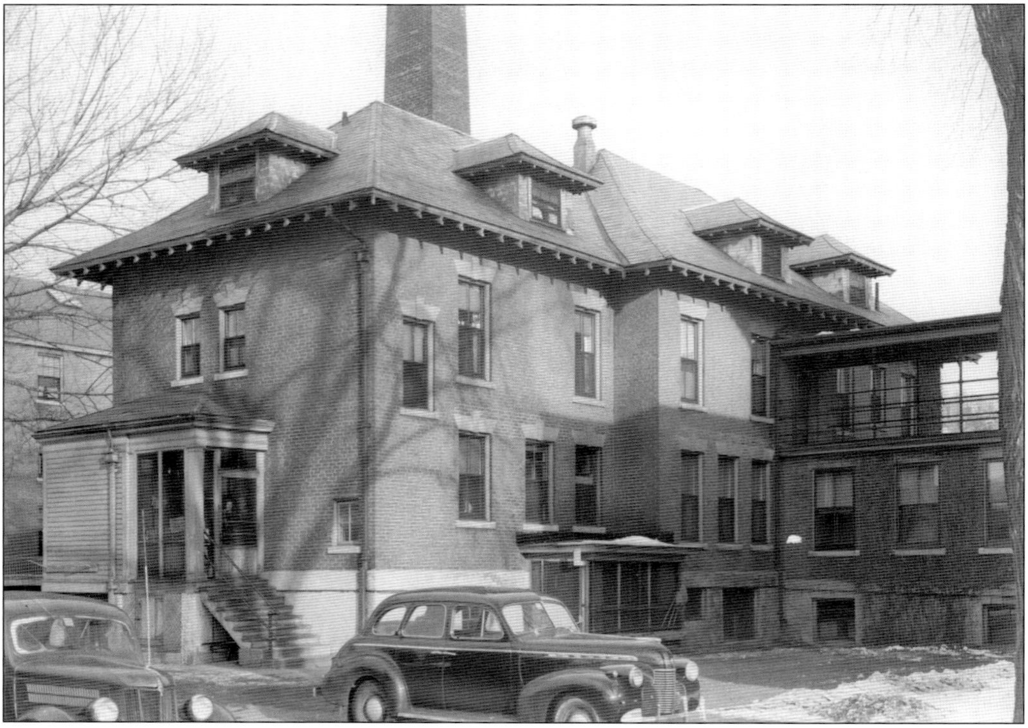

This 1949 photograph shows the back (west and south faces) of the Administration Building. The walkways to the right connected to the South Building. This building would shortly be replaced by the Central Building, constructed with proceeds of the 1945–1949 capital campaign.

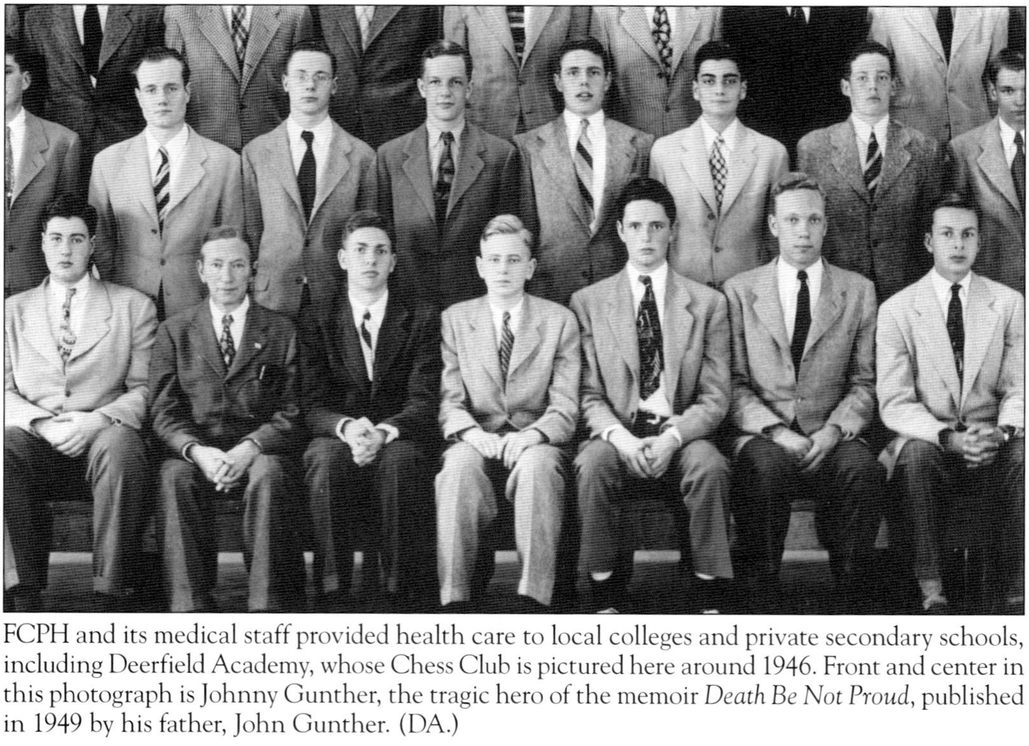

FCPH and its medical staff provided health care to local colleges and private secondary schools, including Deerfield Academy, whose Chess Club is pictured here around 1946. Front and center in this photograph is Johnny Gunther, the tragic hero of the memoir *Death Be Not Proud*, published in 1949 by his father, John Gunther. (DA.)

In the book and later movie, FCPH neurologist Dr. Joseph Hahn (pictured), delivers the diagnosis of glioblastoma, which will ultimately be fatal. *Death Be Not Proud* details Johnny's courageous struggle with his terminal diagnosis and his efforts to graduate from Deerfield Academy, which he accomplished in June 1947.

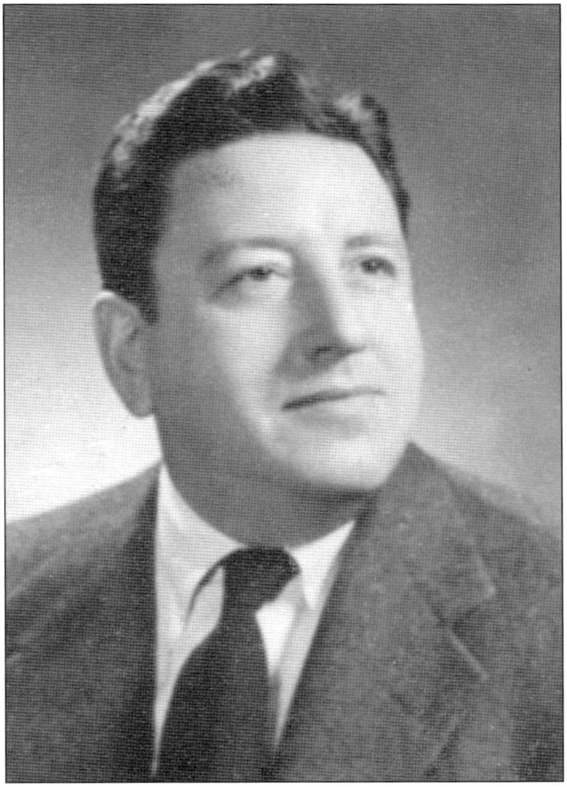

Ginny Short, a laboratory technician, is pictured in 1949. Before the advent of automated blood analyzers, laboratory diagnosis involved hand-mixing of reagents and timed observation of color changes to samples. (Courtesy of Carol Benoit.)

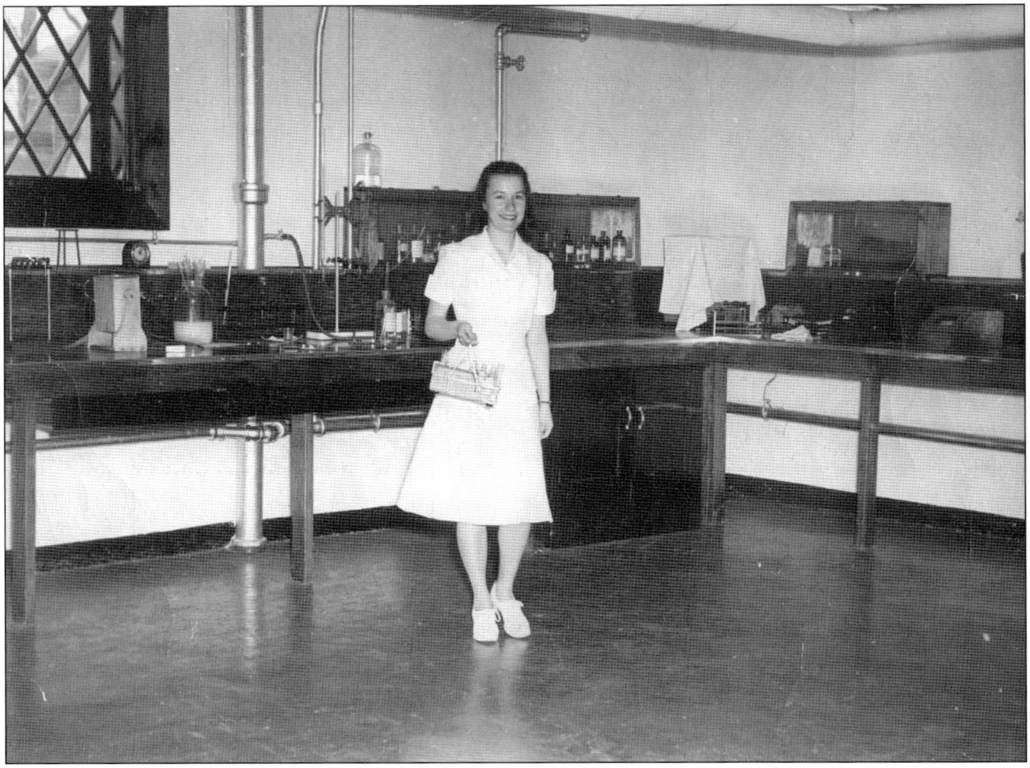

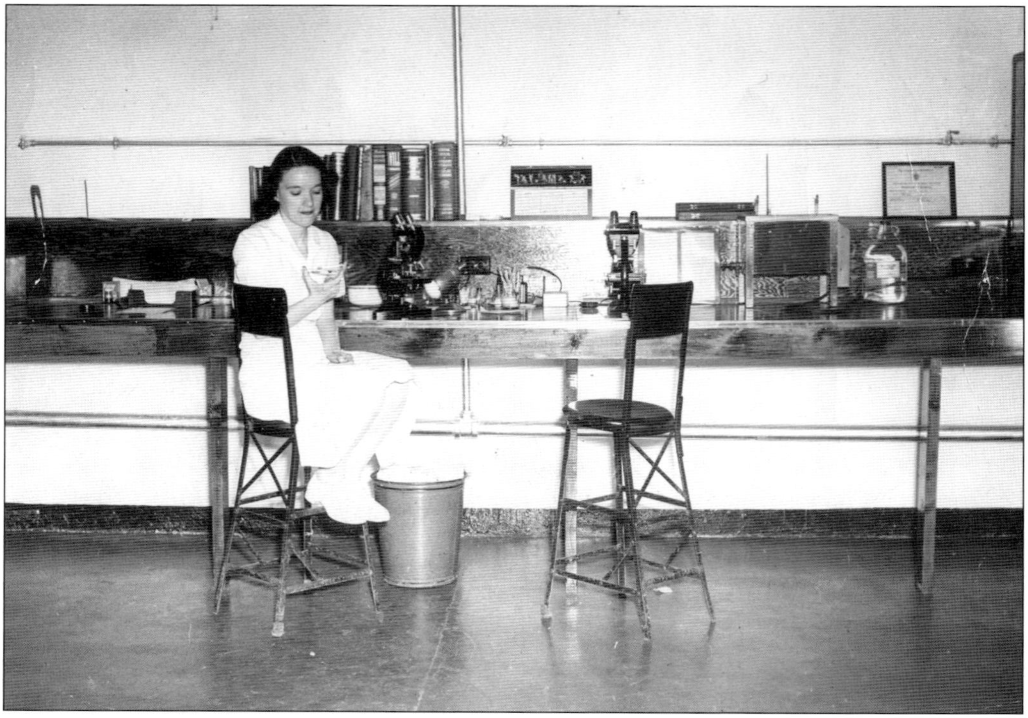

Claire Mercier Coogan is pictured in the laboratory in 1949. She is holding a glass plate about to be examined under one of the two microscopes. (Courtesy of Carol Benoit.)

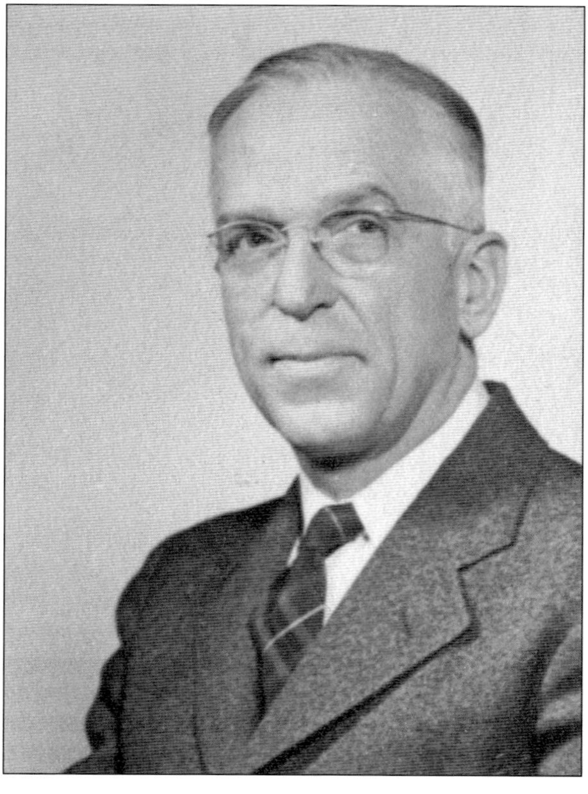

Philip Dudley Woodbridge was an anesthesiologist, innovator, inventor, and pacifist. He studied at the Mayo Clinic and practiced at Lahey Clinic in Boston before joining the FCPH staff in 1949, where he remained until his retirement in 1967. Prior to World War II, most anesthesia was delivered by nurse anesthetists, but advances in technology and surgical procedures between the wars had created a greater role for physician anesthesiologists. Woodbridge was an early innovator in anesthesia safety, advocating for carbon dioxide absorbers, spinal anesthesia, and safer anesthetics, and developing a non-collapsing endotracheal tube. He was also a founding member of the editorial board of the journal *Anesthesiology* and chairman of the Section on Anesthesiology for the American Medical Association in 1963. An accomplished violist, he also played in the Greenfield Symphony Orchestra.

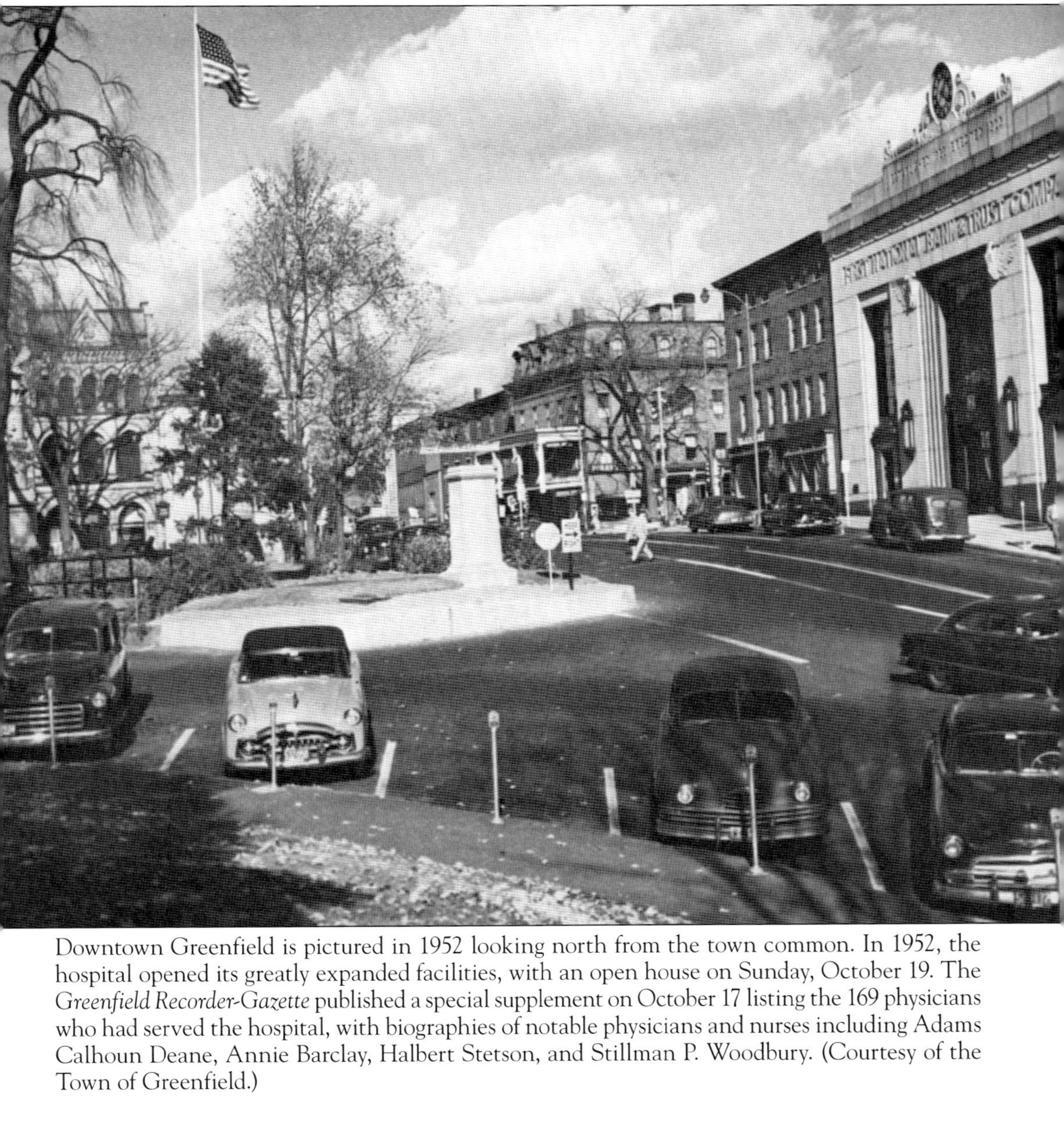

Downtown Greenfield is pictured in 1952 looking north from the town common. In 1952, the hospital opened its greatly expanded facilities, with an open house on Sunday, October 19. The *Greenfield Recorder-Gazette* published a special supplement on October 17 listing the 169 physicians who had served the hospital, with biographies of notable physicians and nurses including Adams Calhoun Deane, Annie Barclay, Halbert Stetson, and Stillman P. Woodbury. (Courtesy of the Town of Greenfield.)

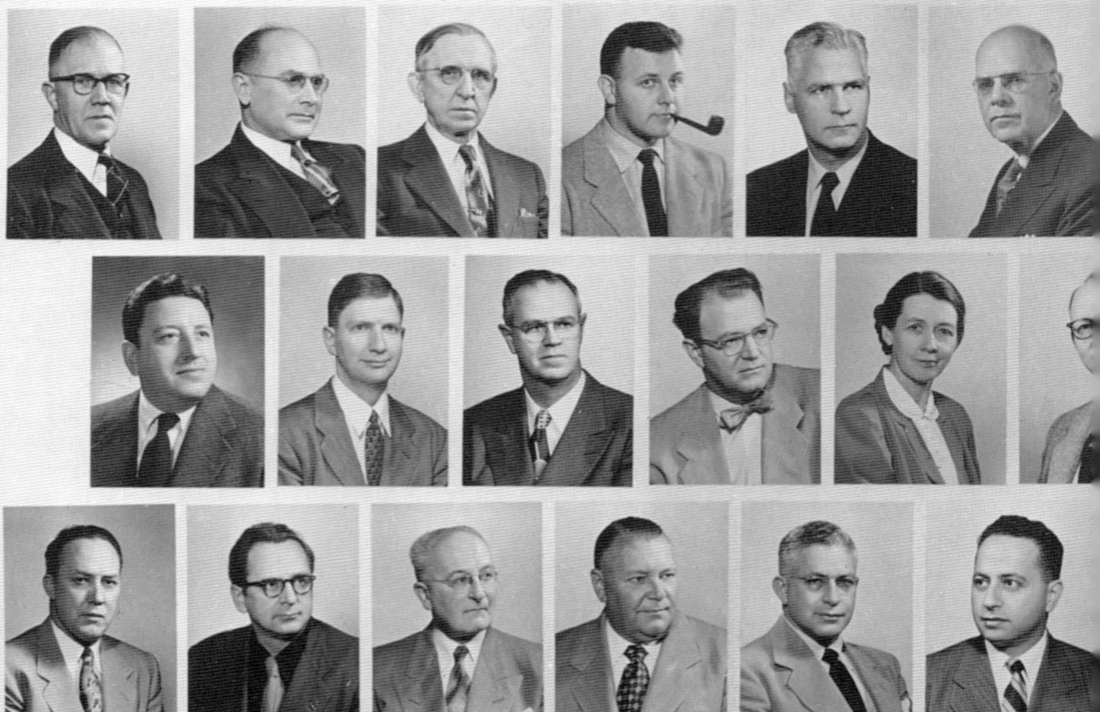

MEDICAL STAFF-19
FRANKLIN COUNTY PUBLIC HOSP

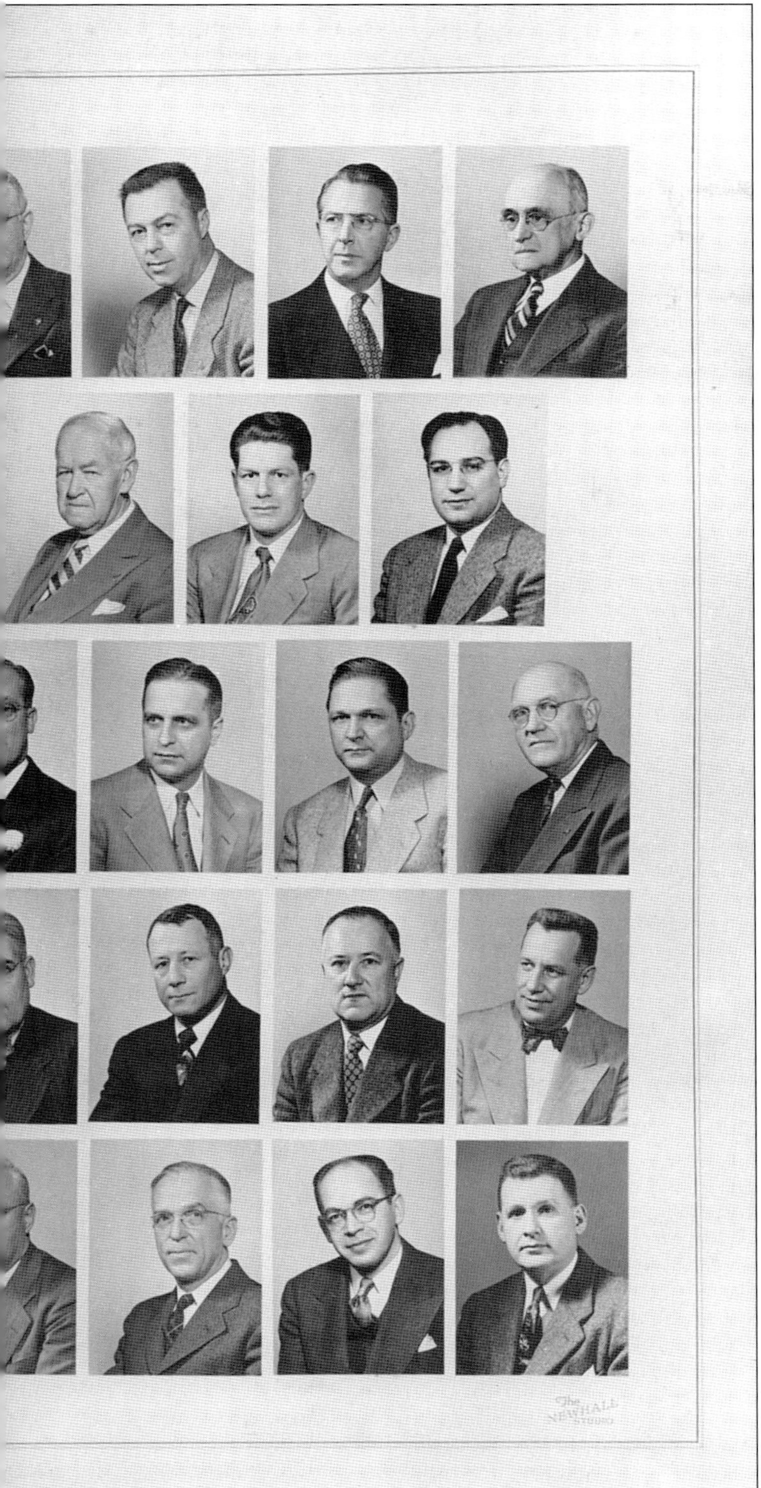

Franklin County Public Hospital's medical staff is pictured in 1952. In the early postwar years, specialists began to arrive, augmenting the capabilities of the hospital to provide cutting-edge care.

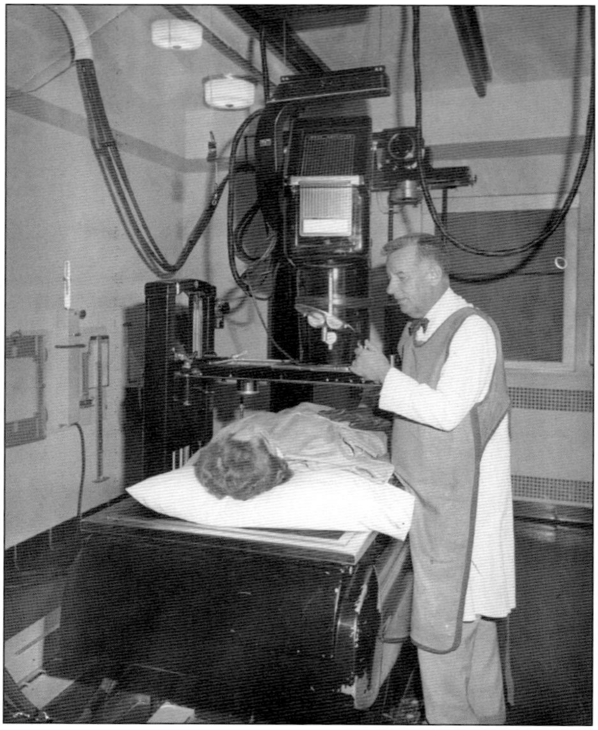

Dr. Donald P. Ham joined the FCPH staff in 1947, becoming the first fulltime radiologist. He is pictured adjusting an X-ray machine above a patient. His right hand is enclosed in a lead glove, and he is wearing a lead apron to shield against repeated radiation exposure.

FCPH physicians were expected to participate in the training of nurses and radiology technologists. Dr. Ham is seated in front of a light box used to read films; four students are looking at details on abdominal/spine films and skull X-rays. Today, film has been replaced by electronic images. FCPH ran a school of radiologic technology from 1922 until it was phased out in 1947 as hospital-based training was replaced by community college programs.

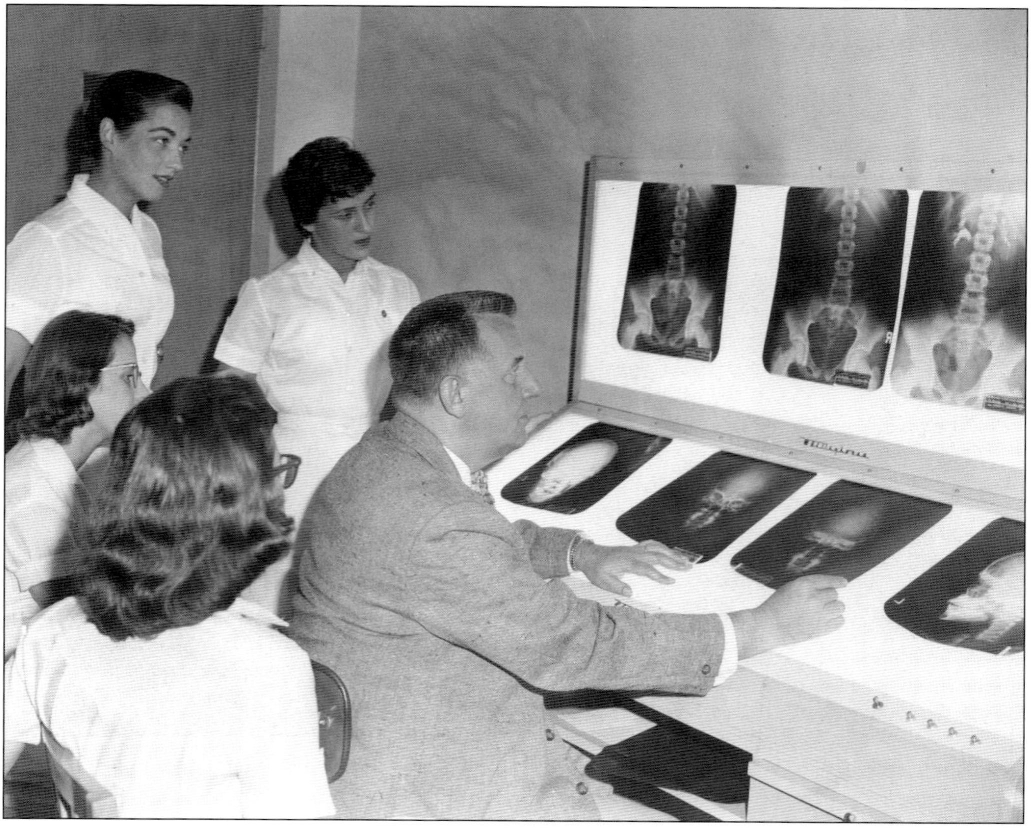

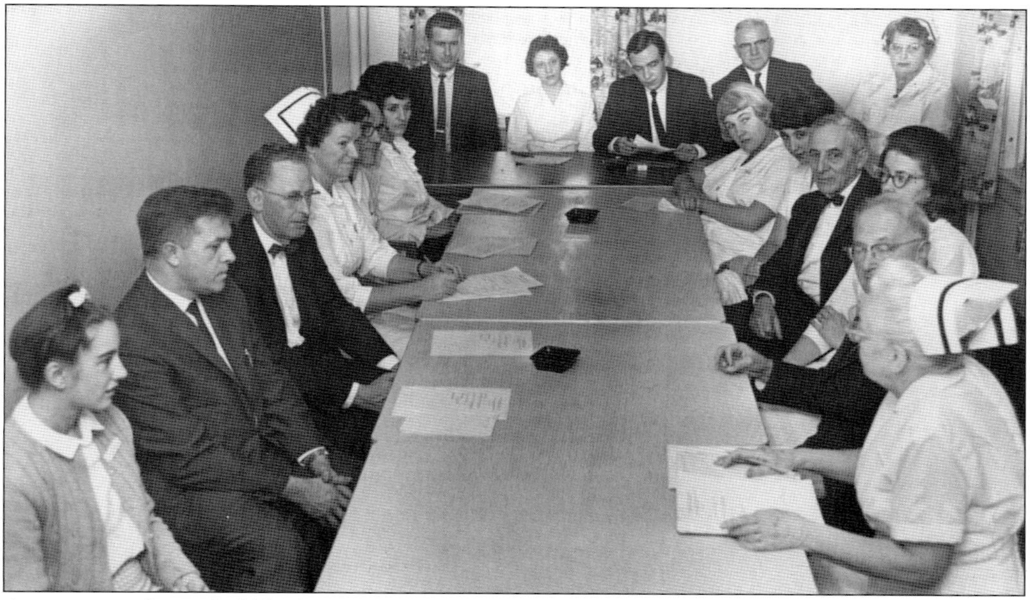

A meeting is being held by hospital members around 1966. Identified are, in no particular order, Mrs. Poirier, Dr. Adler, Dr. Nobel, Martha Seward, William Christenson, Wally Houston, and Barb Mathews. Meetings such as this were held on a regular basis and may have involved a discussion over a patient's care.

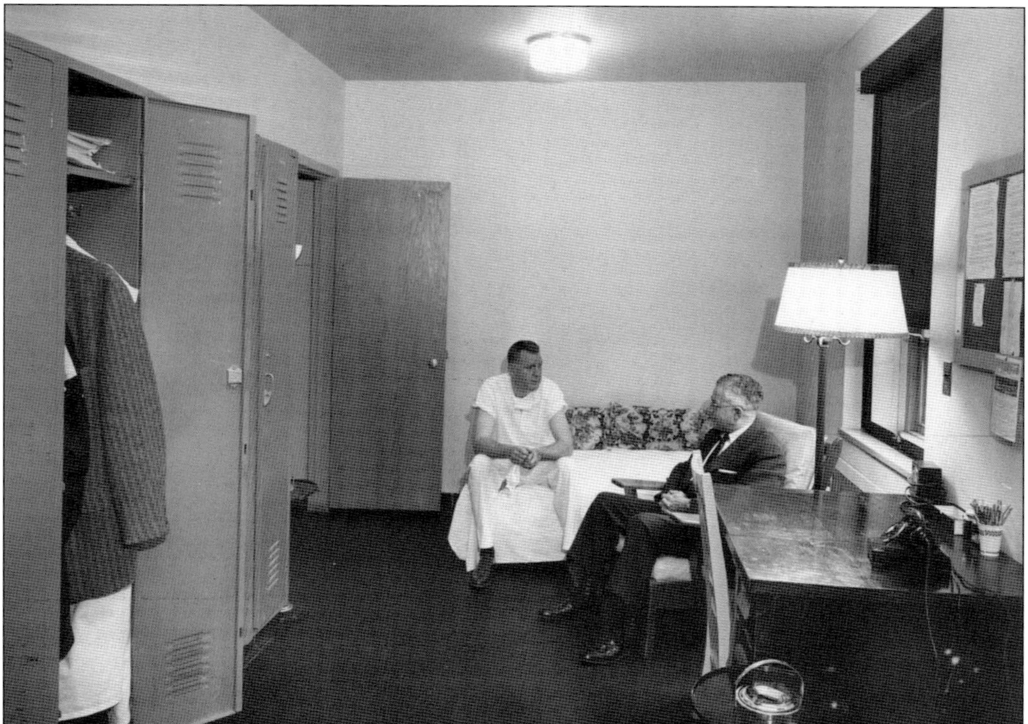

The Physician's On-Call Room is pictured around 1966. The two physicians are unidentified. Sleeping facilities were provided for surgeons and obstetricians who were on call for emergency procedures or deliveries.

VISITING HOURS

Medical & Surgical floors	10 a.m. to 8:30 p.m.
Maternity floor	2 p.m. to 3:30 p.m. 7 p.m. to 8:30 p.m.
Pediatric rooms	10 a.m. to 12 a.m. 2 p.m. to 7 p.m.
Nursery	3 p.m. to 3:30 p.m. 7 p.m. to 7:30 p.m.
Ambulatory Care	10 a.m. to 10 p.m.

Intense Care Unit — Visits limited to 5 minutes.

Only two visitors to each patient.

Children under 14 may not visit patients.

Hospital experience has shown that these requirements are in the best interests of good patient care.

THE FRANKLIN COUNTY PUBLIC HOSPITAL

☆

Schedule of Hospital Charges

OCTOBER 1, 1963

This FCPH schedule of hospital charges is from October 1963. Visiting hours were from 10:00 a.m. to 8:30 p.m. on medical and surgical floors but were more limited on the maternity floor and pediatrics. Intensive Care Unit visits were limited to five minutes, and children under the age of 14 were not permitted to visit at all.

ROUTINE CHARGES

Private

A	~~$33.00~~	35.50
B	~~$32.00~~	34.50
D	~~$30.00~~	32.50
E	~~$29.00~~	31.50

Semi-Private

2-bed A	~~$28.50~~	30.50
2-bed B	~~$27.00~~	29
3-bed	~~$27.00~~	29
4-bed	~~$26.00~~	28
Intense Care Unit	~~$42.00~~	45
Ambulatory Care Unit	~~$18.00~~	19.50
Pediatric	~~$21.00~~	23

Ward

5-bed	~~$23.00~~	26
7-bed	~~$22.50~~	25.50

Ward accommodations are reserved for Public Assistance patients.

Maternity

Private	$28.50
2-bed	$24.50
3-bed	$22.50
4-bed	$21.50

Nursery

Nursing Baby	~~$10.00~~	11.50
Bottle Baby	~~$12.00~~	13.50
After Mother's Discharge	~~$15.00~~	16.50

Sanderson Evaluation Unit #10

Routine charges listed are for room, board and 24-hour nursing care. They do not include doctors' or private nurses' fees. Private nurses are not utilized in the intense care unit.

OTHER CHARGES

Operating room, delivery room, anesthesia, x-rays, laboratory, drugs, medical supplies and other services ordered by your doctor are not included in the room rates. These other charges presently average $11.50 a day but may be higher or lower depending on your need for special services as determined by your doctor.

GENERAL INFORMATION

Pediatric rooms generally are for children of 14 years and under.

Assignment to intensive care or ambulatory care unit is on doctors' orders only.

Price increases were hand-edited on this 1963 brochure and reflected substantial increases for the day. Room rates in 2015 for a semi-private room are $1,050; the five- and seven-bed wards are long gone. A similar brochure from 1966 reflects that semi-private room rates had increased to $37.50 per day.

Seven

The Spokes

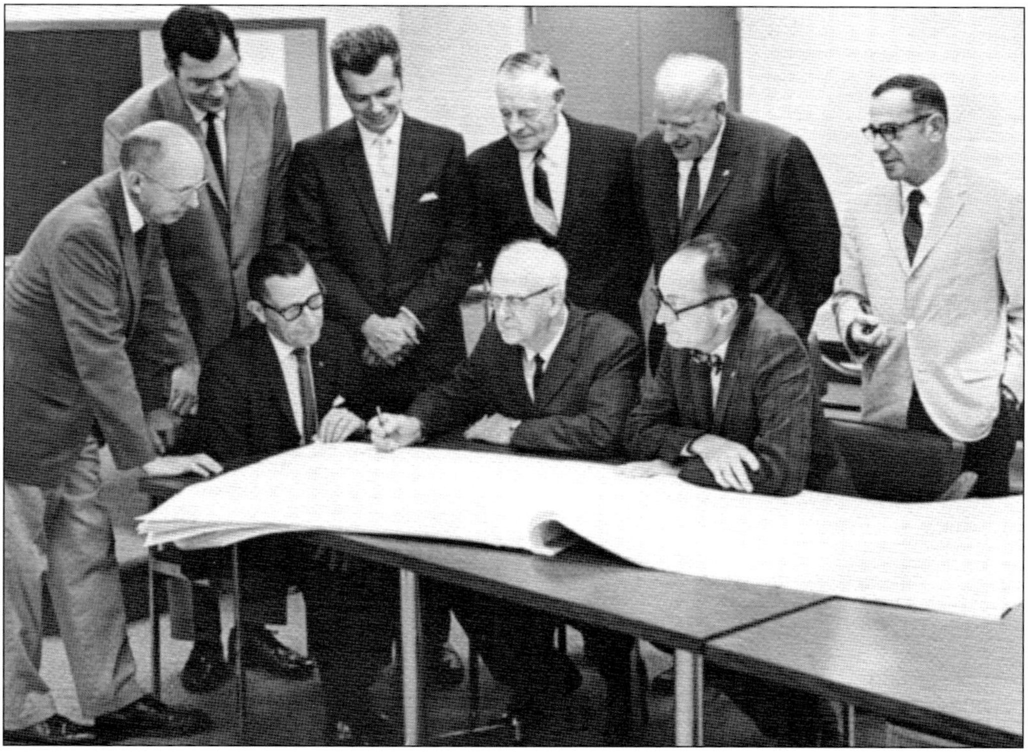

Committee members look over early plans in 1962. Standing, from left to right, are Dr. Jim Sinisger, Bill Zwempke, Don Lorenz, Darius Kelley, Andy Waite, and Simon Cohen. Those seated are thought to be Richard Lyman, architect Sherman Morss, and hospital director Bright Dornblaster.

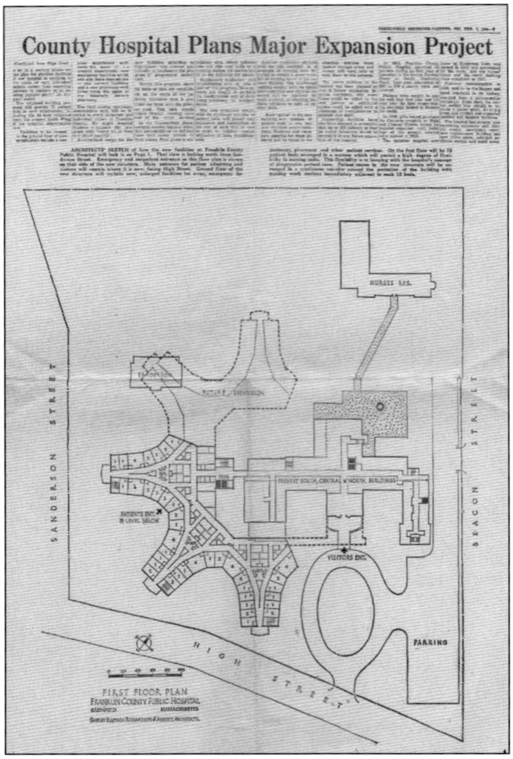

Initial plans from the architectural firm of Shepley Bulfinch Richardson & Abbott called for construction of three spokes and allowed for future expansion on the site of the Sanderson building, the former isolation hospital. Patient rooms lined the exterior walls to maximize light and views and were built as a mixture of single, double, and four-bed wards. Nursing stations and support services occupied interior spaces. The project was designed in phases to allow for eventual removal of the original South Building.

This plan more closely represents what was built, with the axes of the spokes rotated slightly to preserve the Sanderson building. The construction sequences were altered to first build Spokes II, III, and IV, and a radiology suite has been added.

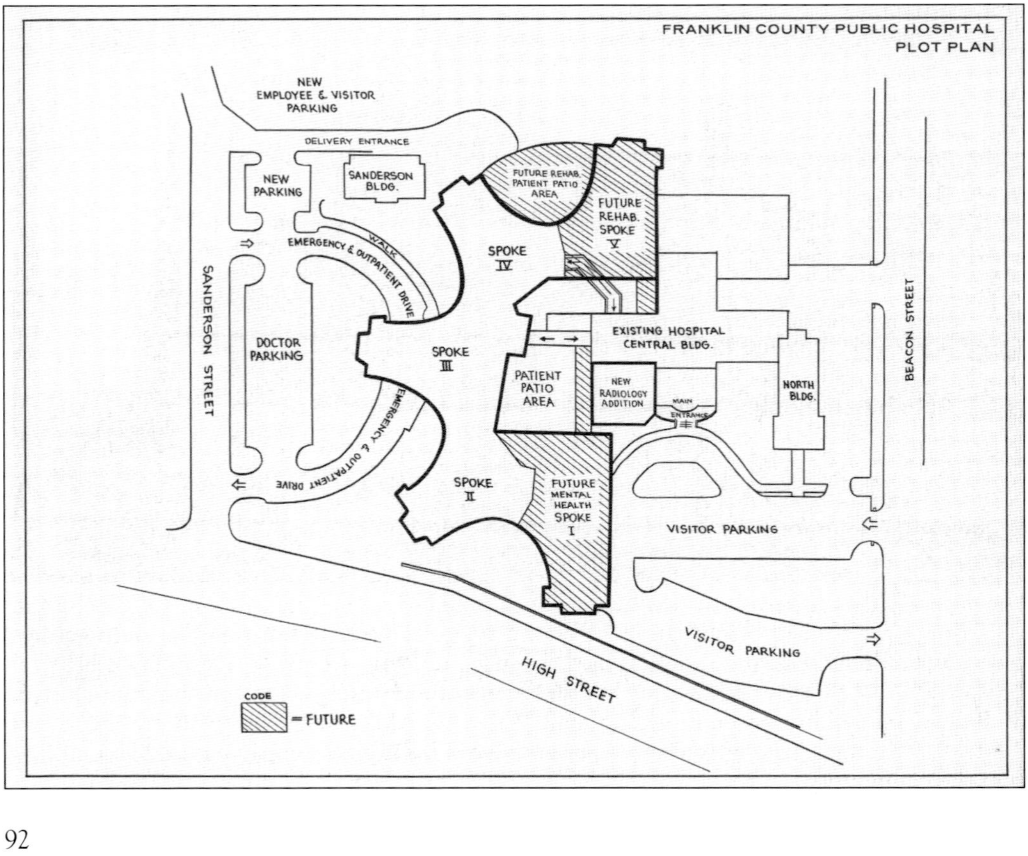

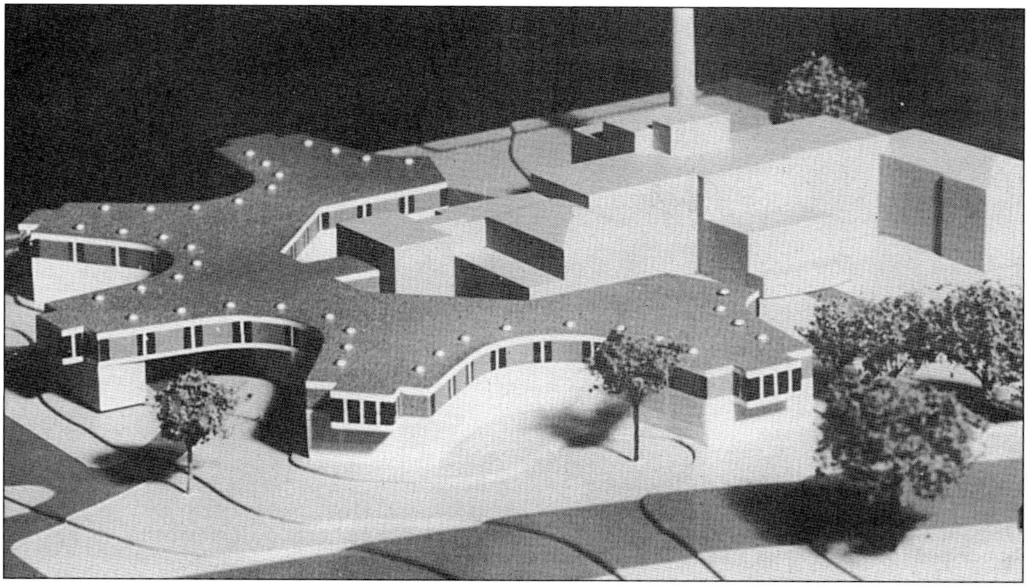

This architect's model of the future hospital shows five spokes completed. In this vision, the 1910-vintage South Wing was to be preserved, a decision that was later reversed owing to issues with the age and wood-frame construction of the original hospital building. Modern building codes no longer permit housing inpatients in wood-frame structures.

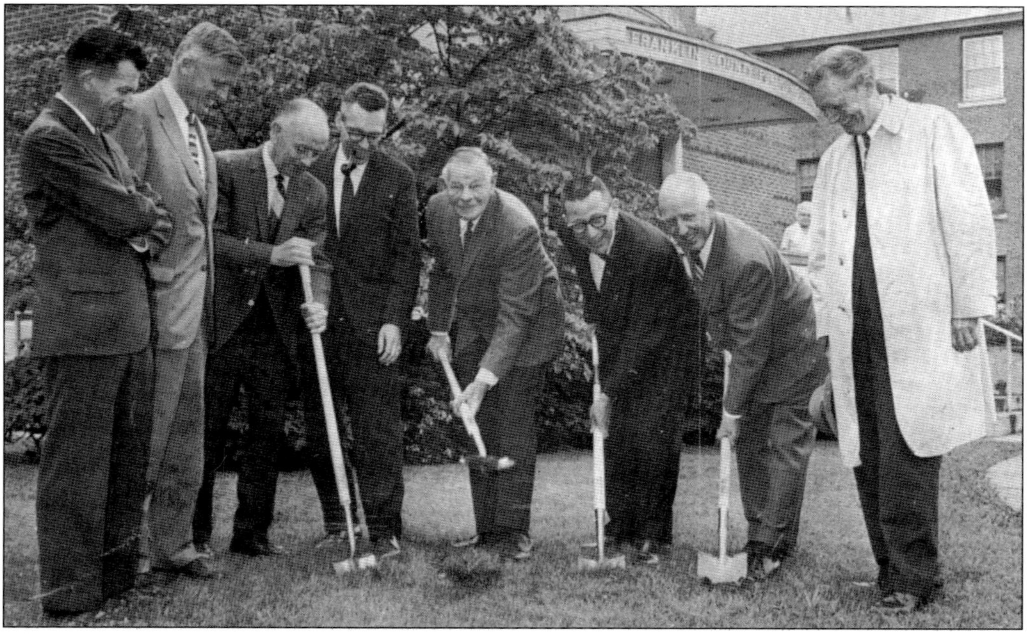

The groundbreaking ceremony for the new Spokes addition was held on June 10, 1966. From left to right are Russell Bishop and Sherman Morse, representatives from the architectural firm; Dr. Aaron W. Newton, hospital medical staff president; Bright M. Dornblaser, hospital director; Paul W. Shores, representing John W. Haigis, fund-raising campaign chairman; Joseph W. Ballard Jr., building committee chairman; Allen W. Abercrombie, hospital president; and Daniel J. O'Connell, general contract representative. This capital campaign raised $1.5 million from the community.

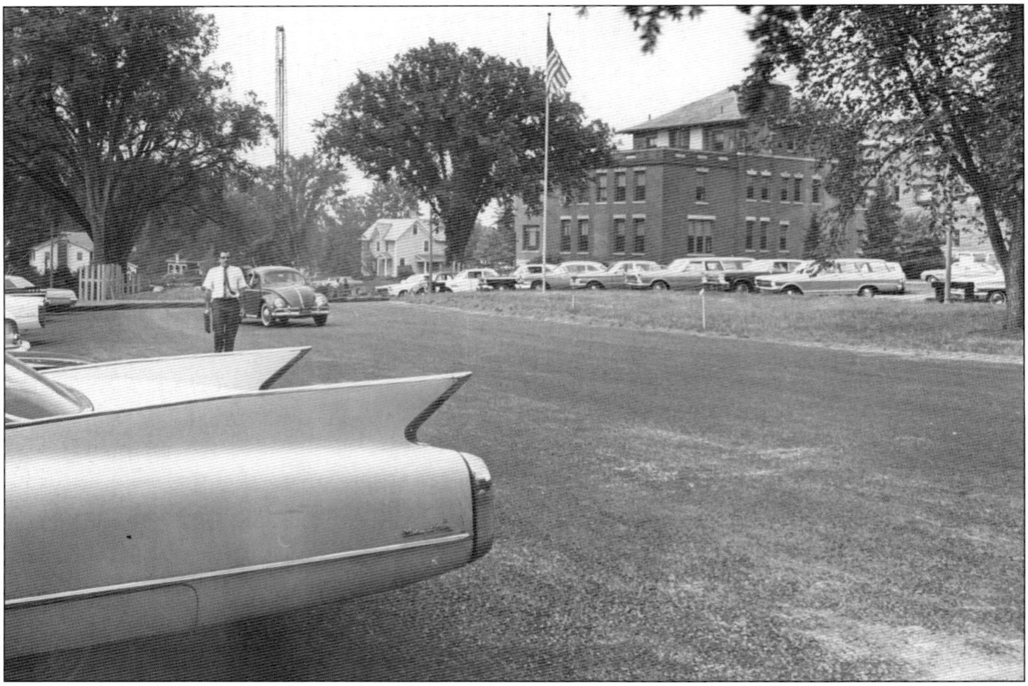

This photograph, taken on August 11, 1966, shows a pile driver emerging at the Spokes construction site to the left of the South Building. The 1960 Cadillac in the foreground sports impressive tail fins.

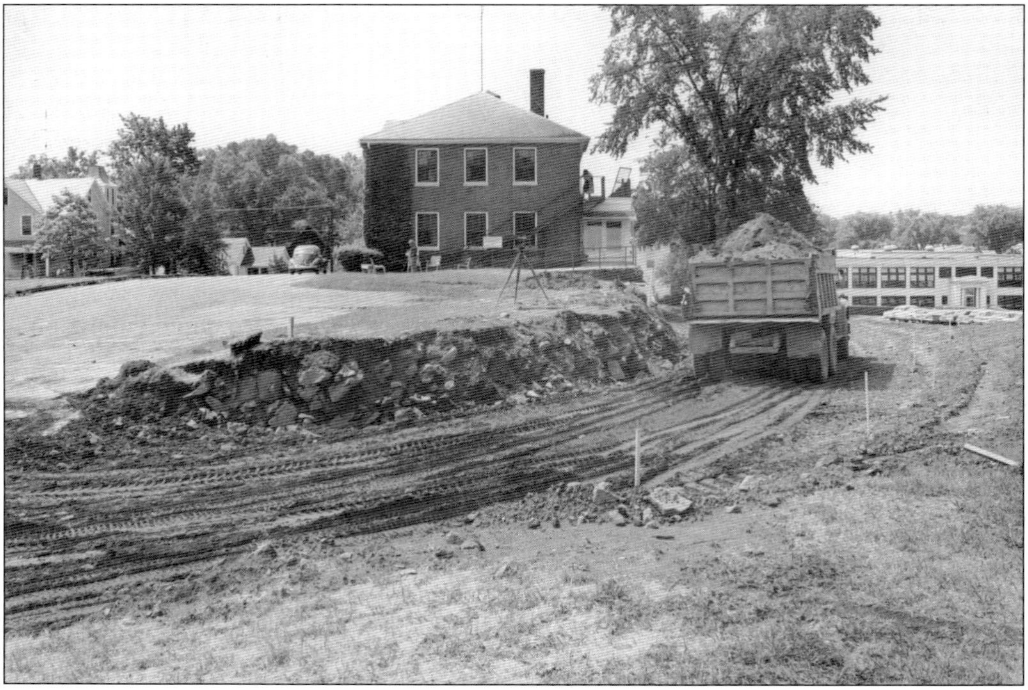

Construction has begun on July 21, 1966. The Sanderson building is in the center, and the Greenfield Tap and Die (GTD) headquarters is to the right of the dump truck. The GTD building today houses outpatient services for BFMC and the Baystate Health Northern Region.

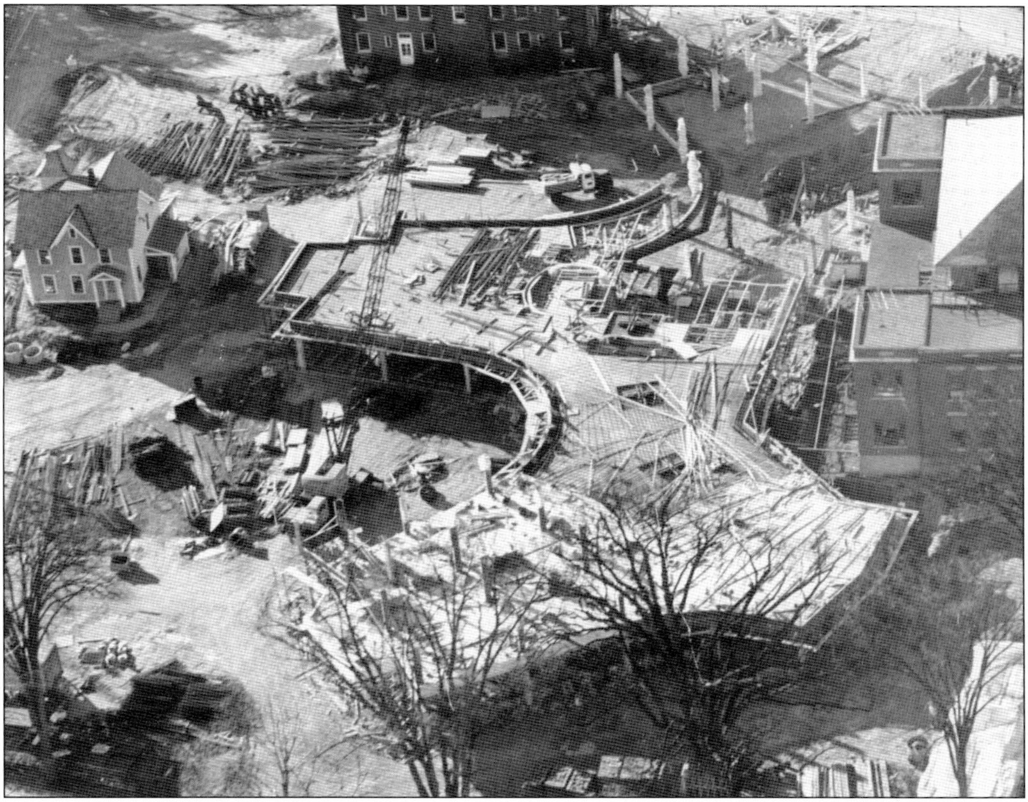

This aerial view from 1967 shows construction in progress for Spokes II, III, and IV. The South Building, to the right, was still in use for patient care, as was the Sanderson building at the top.

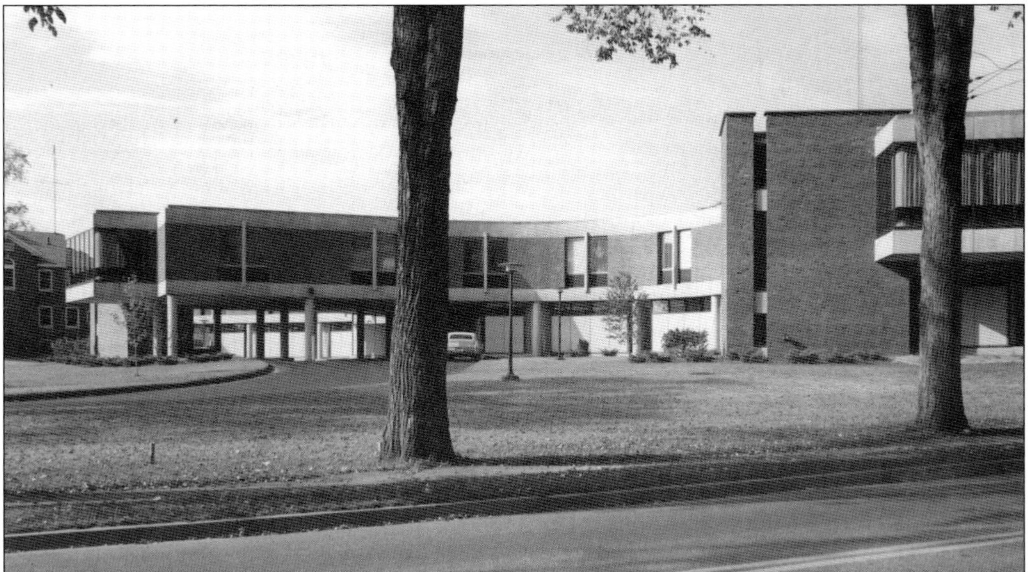

This postcard view shows the completed Spoke III. As originally built, this spoke incorporated carport access to the Emergency Room on the ground floor. Subsequent growth of the Emergency Department claimed this space and altered the sweeping design of the original structure.

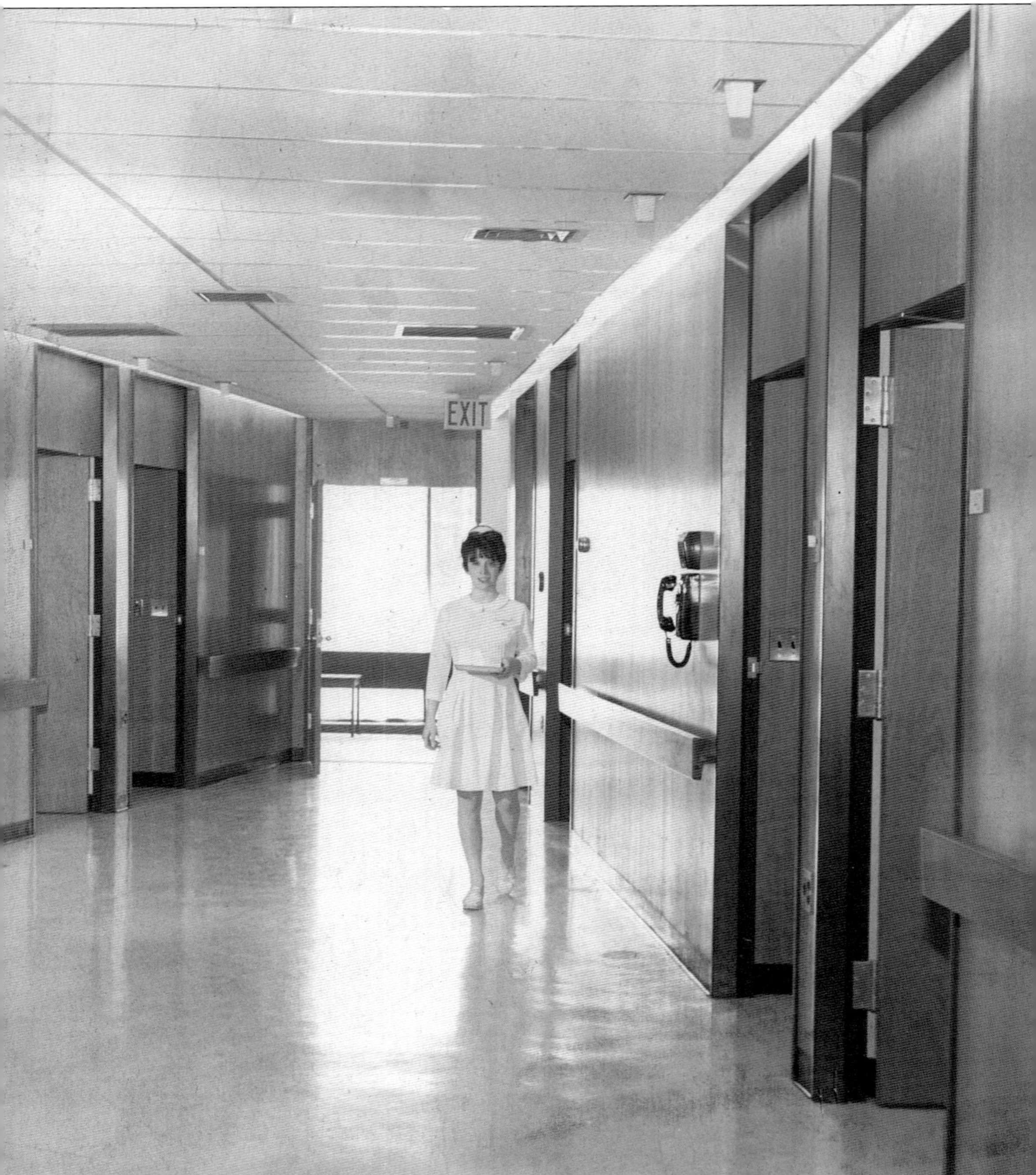

This interior view of Spoke V dates from 1970 or 1971. Spoke V was mothballed in the mid-2000s but reopened in 2015 to accommodate an increased census at BFMC. It is the only spoke that has not been extensively remodeled since construction. In the 1968 dedication ceremony, it was stated that "a new Franklin County Public Hospital will rise and stand as a living, life-giving memorial to the people who have given of themselves and their resources to create it."

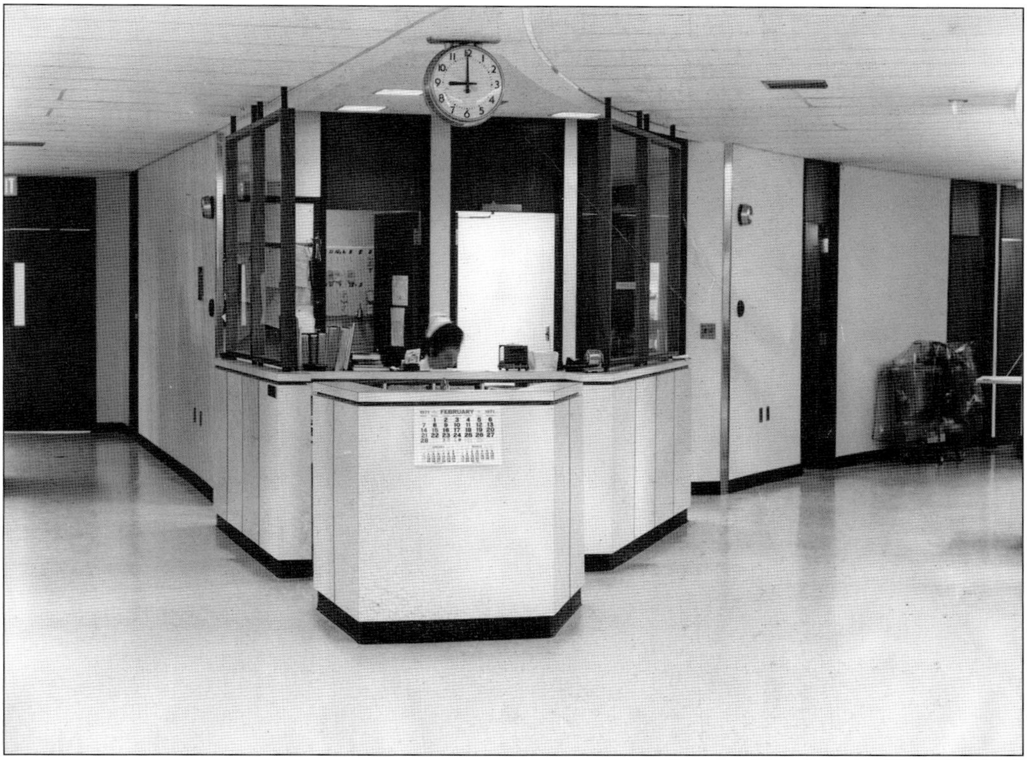

The nursing station in Spoke V is pictured in February 1971. The spokes were designed to provide line-of-sight from the nursing station to each patient room. Medication and supply rooms were provided in the internal areas behind the desk, while exterior walls were preserved for patient rooms.

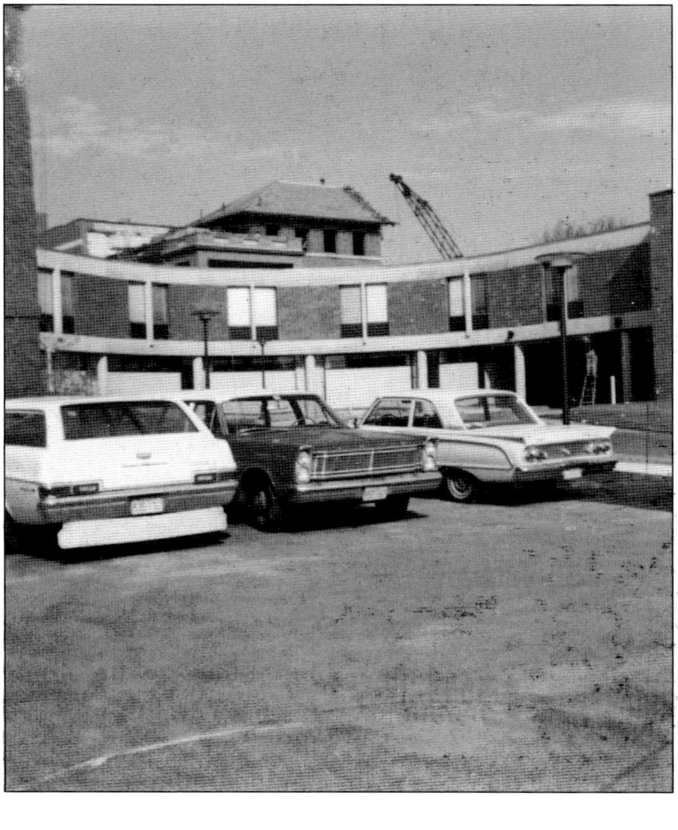

By the winter of 1968, the first three spokes had been occupied, allowing the South Building to be decommissioned. In this photograph, demolition has already claimed the portion of the building facing High Street, and the rest will soon follow.

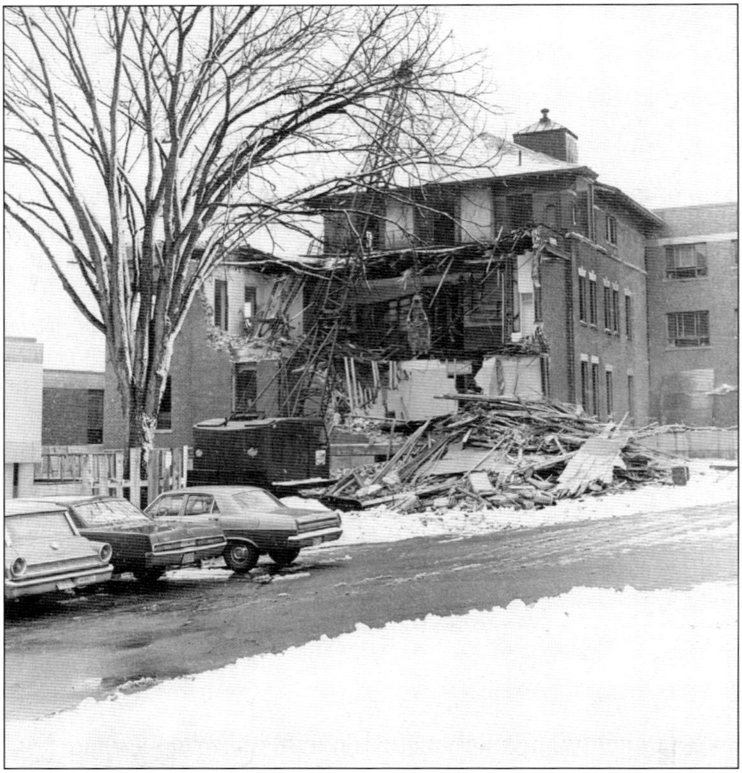

Here is another view of the South Building's demolition, this time from High Street. The space created became the patient patio area bounded by Spokes I, II, and III and a connecting hallway to the Central Building.

The Spokes project was completed in 1970. This diagram shows the completed design and the relative positions of the Sanderson building (near Spoke IV) and the nursing school (to the left of Spoke V).

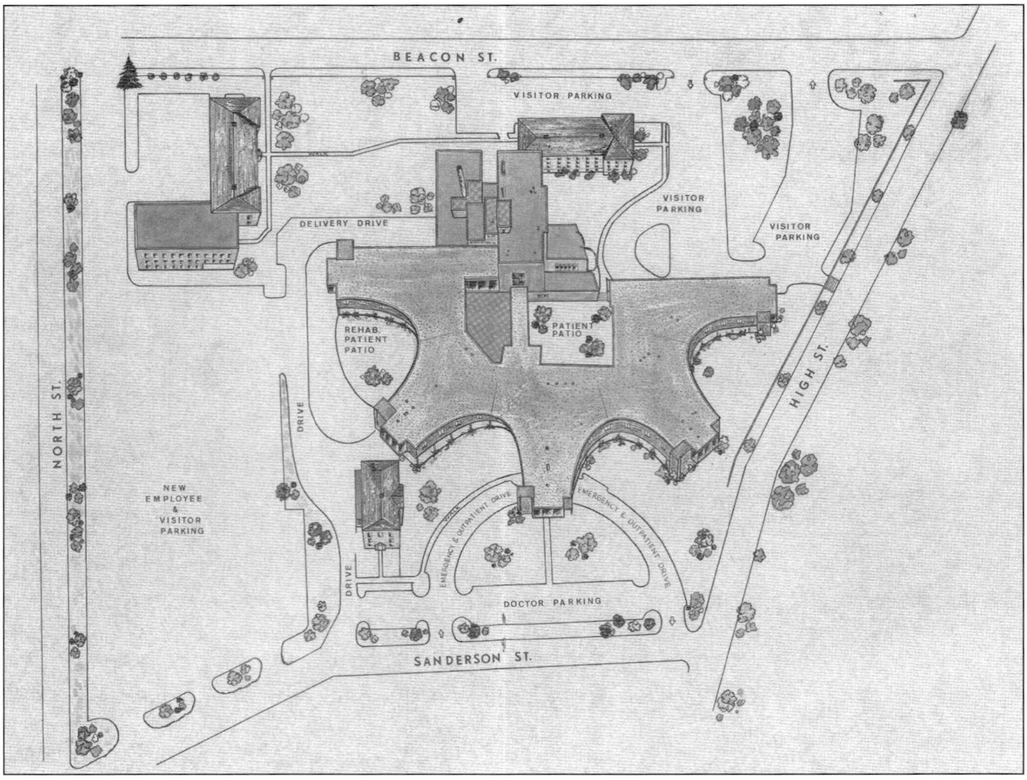

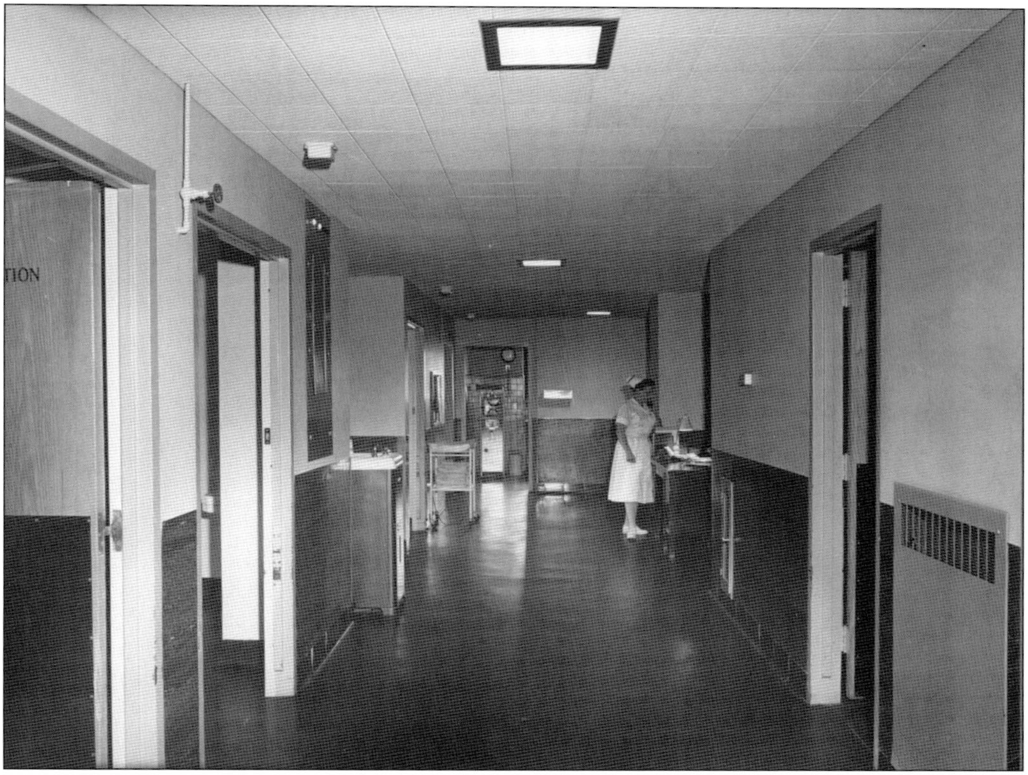

The spokes contained patient rooms; the operating rooms were concentrated in the Central Building after South 3 was decommissioned but before the Russell Building opened in 1975.

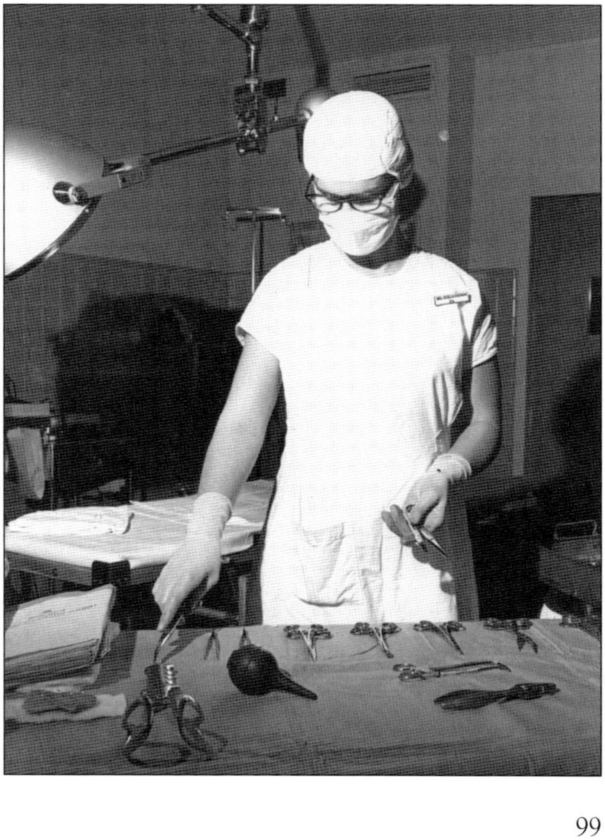

Cecelia Sherman, RN, organizes sterile instruments in this 1968 photograph.

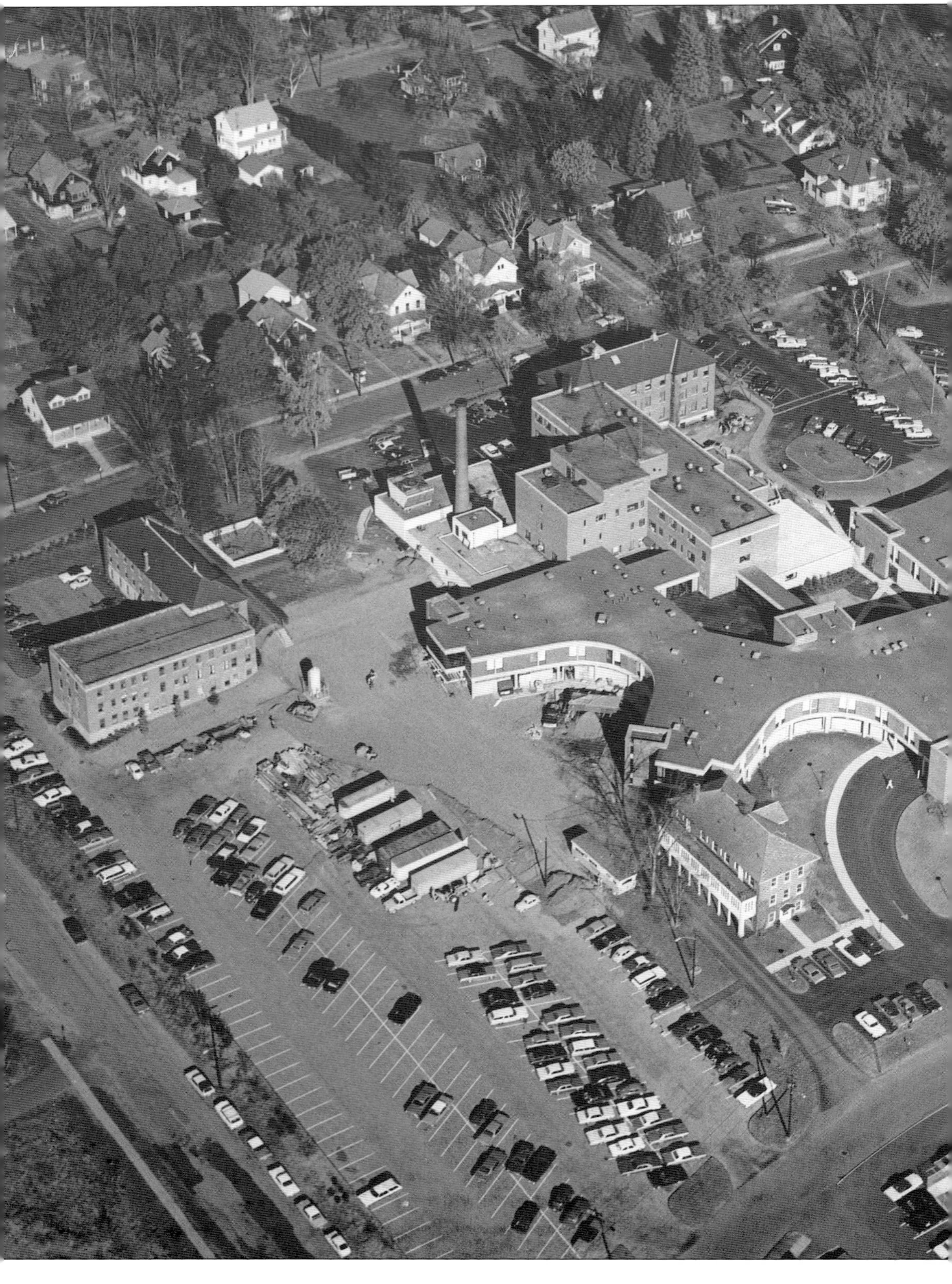

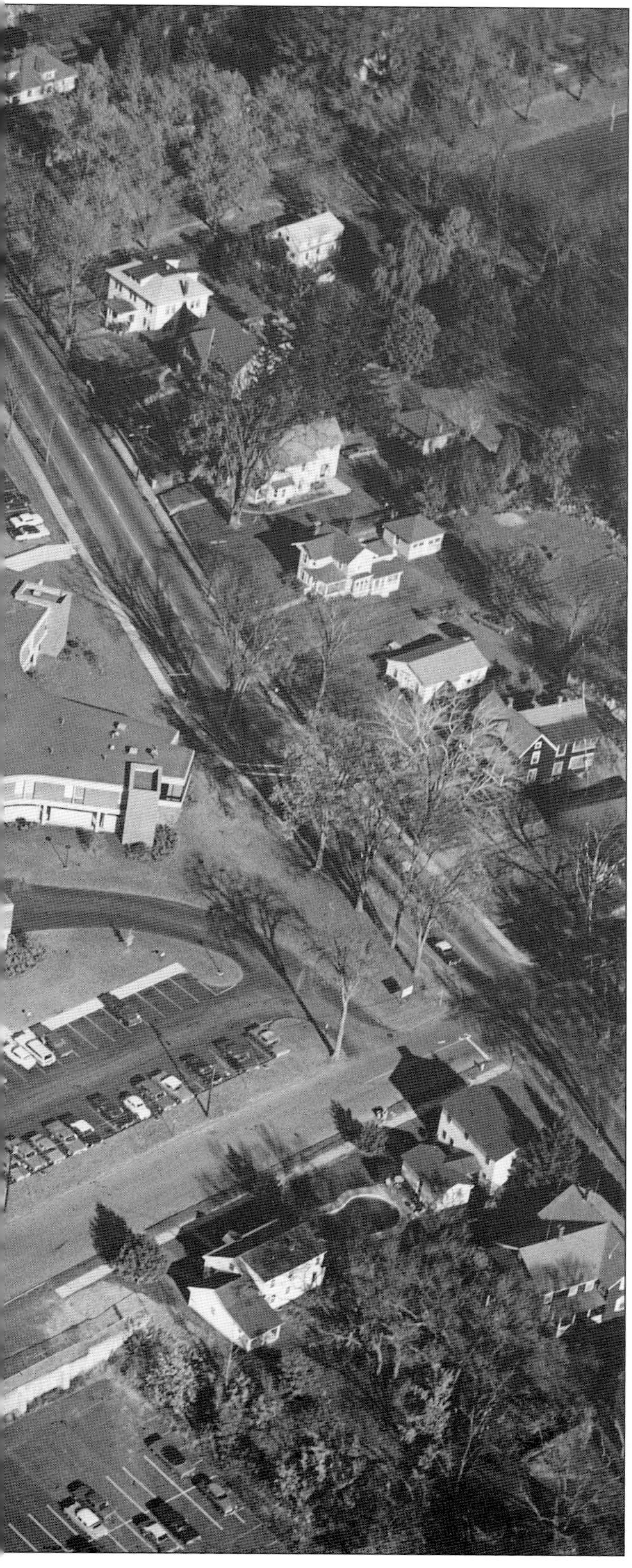

The American Hospital Association featured FCPH as its Modern Hospital of the Month in 1970. This aerial view captures the innovative design. The brick towers towards the end of each spoke contain stairwells, and each spoke had an enclosed sun porch for patients.

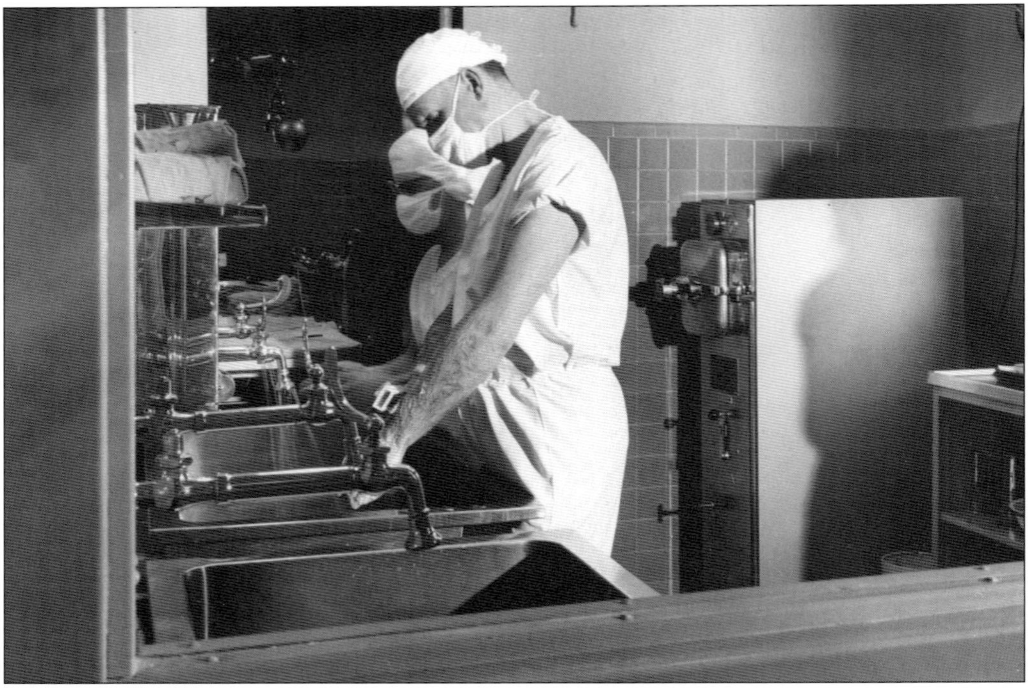

A nurse and physician scrub prior to gloving and gowning. The faucets at the scrub sink are equipped with handles that can be turned with the elbow. The operating room is to the rear. The device to the right is a sterilizer.

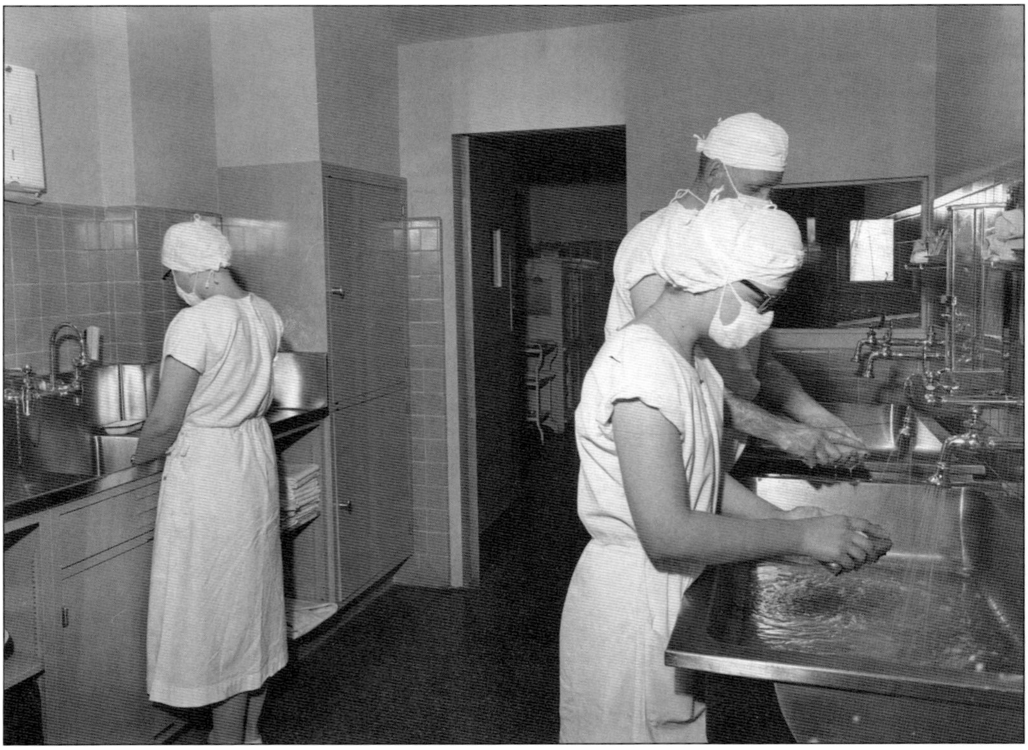

Another view shows the operating suite scrub room seen in the prior image.

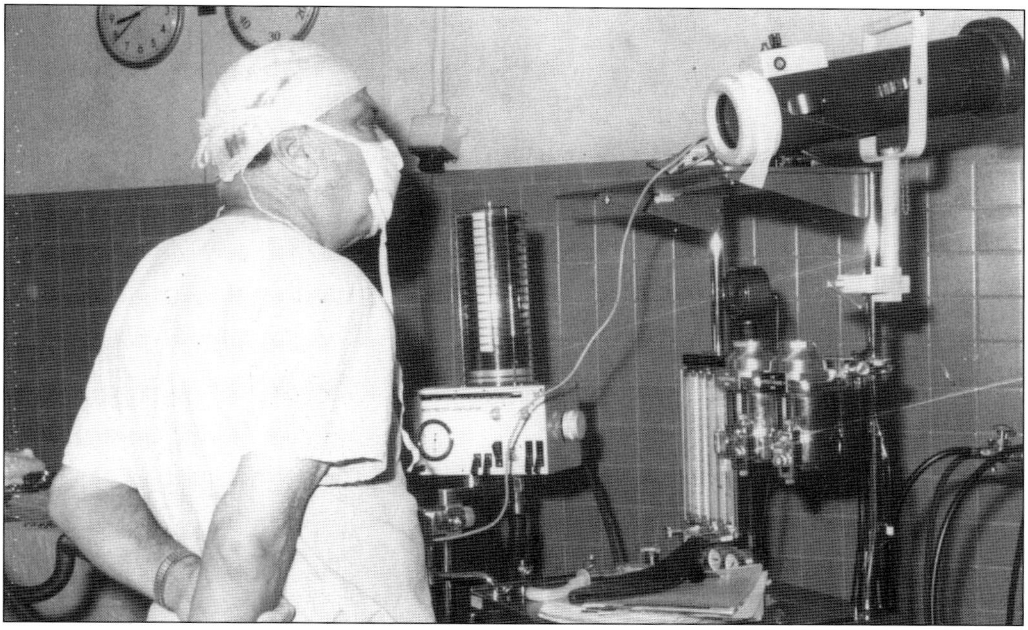

Dr. Julian Nieckoski, anesthesiologist, monitors the patient's electrocardiogram (EKG) on a vintage "bullet" monitor, consisting of a cathode ray tube housed in a cylinder. Under the monitor are vaporizers for the anesthetic agents halothane and penthrane. The vintage ventilator and anesthesia equipment would date this picture to the late 1960s or early 1970s. Penthrane (methoxyflurane) was discovered to be toxic and was replaced by safer alternatives by the mid-1970s.

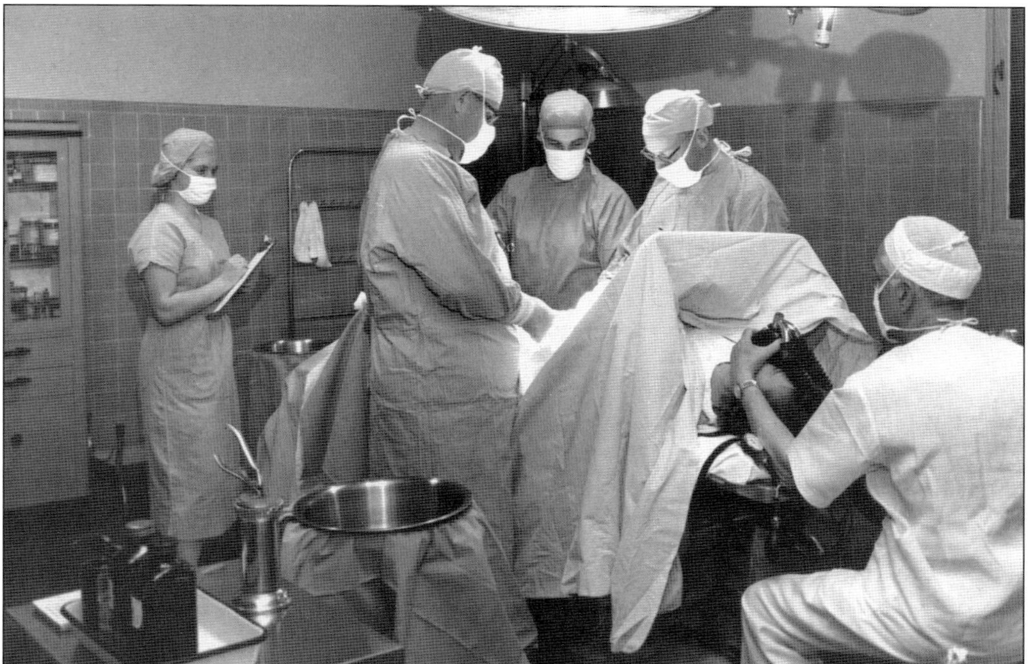

An abdominal surgery is underway in this c. 1968 photograph. The participants are unidentified, but from left to right would be the circulating nurse, the assistant surgeon, the scrub nurse, the surgeon, and the anesthesiologist.

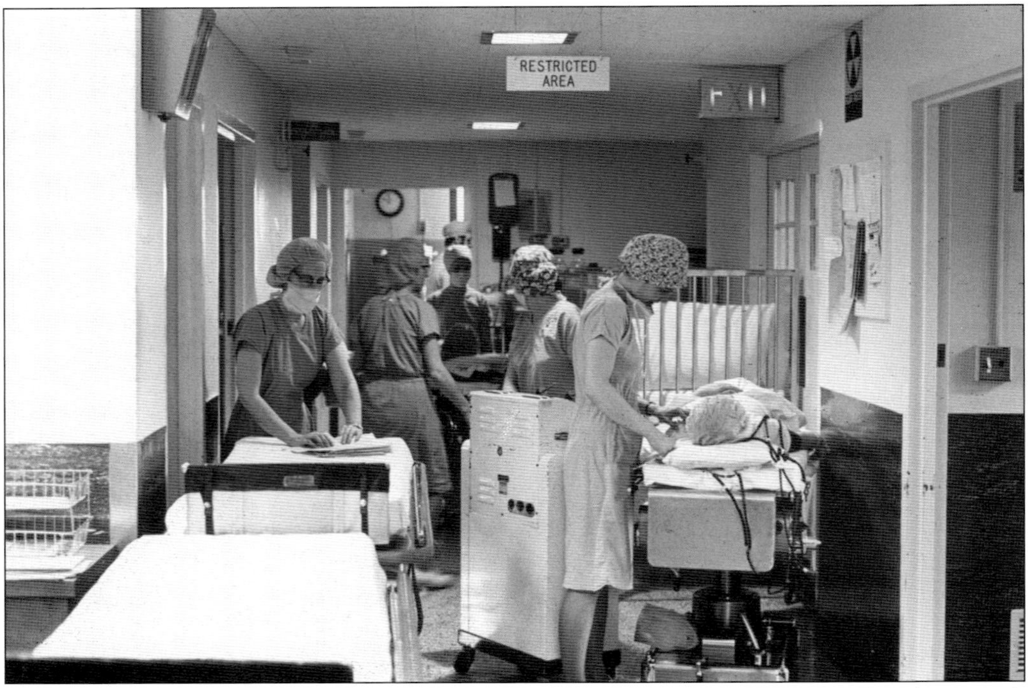

A traffic jam takes place in the operating room corridor in the early 1970s. This photograph documents the crowded conditions in the Central Building's operating rooms, which would be replaced by the Russell Surgical Pavilion in 1975.

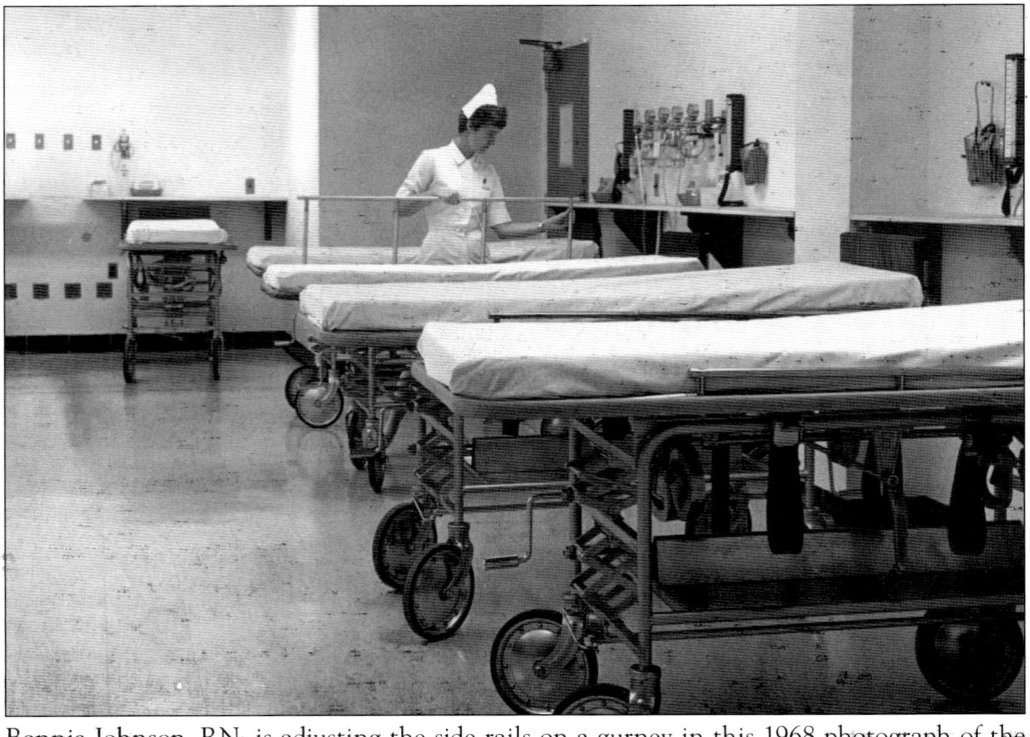

Bonnie Johnson, RN, is adjusting the side rails on a gurney in this 1968 photograph of the preoperative area.

This c. 1970 view is from the anesthesiologist's perspective. The patient's head is this side of the "ether screen," a barrier to delineate the unsterile world of the anesthesiologist from the sterile field where the surgeons are operating.

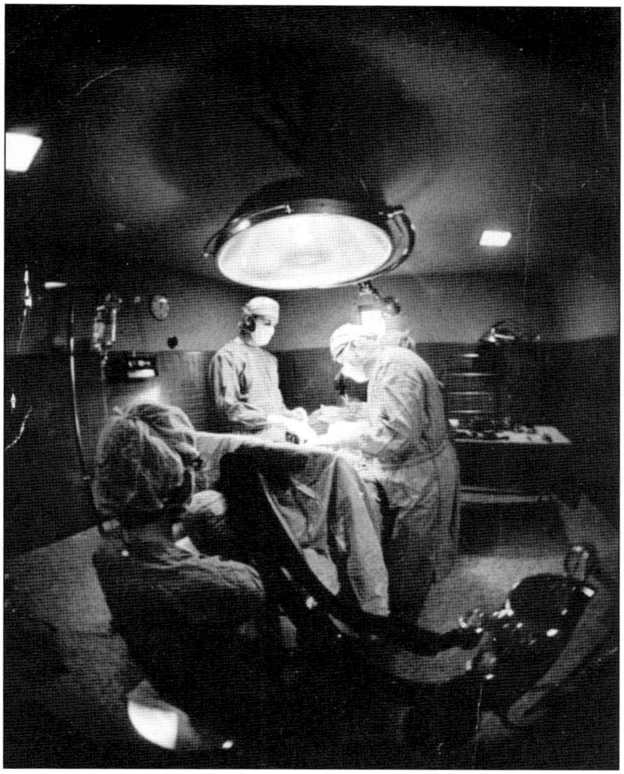

A recovery room in the Central Building is pictured in the early 1970s. Adults and children recovered from anesthesia in the same area, as evidenced by the crib behind the nurses. Today, the term "recovery room" has been replaced by Post-Anesthesia Recovery Unit (PACU).

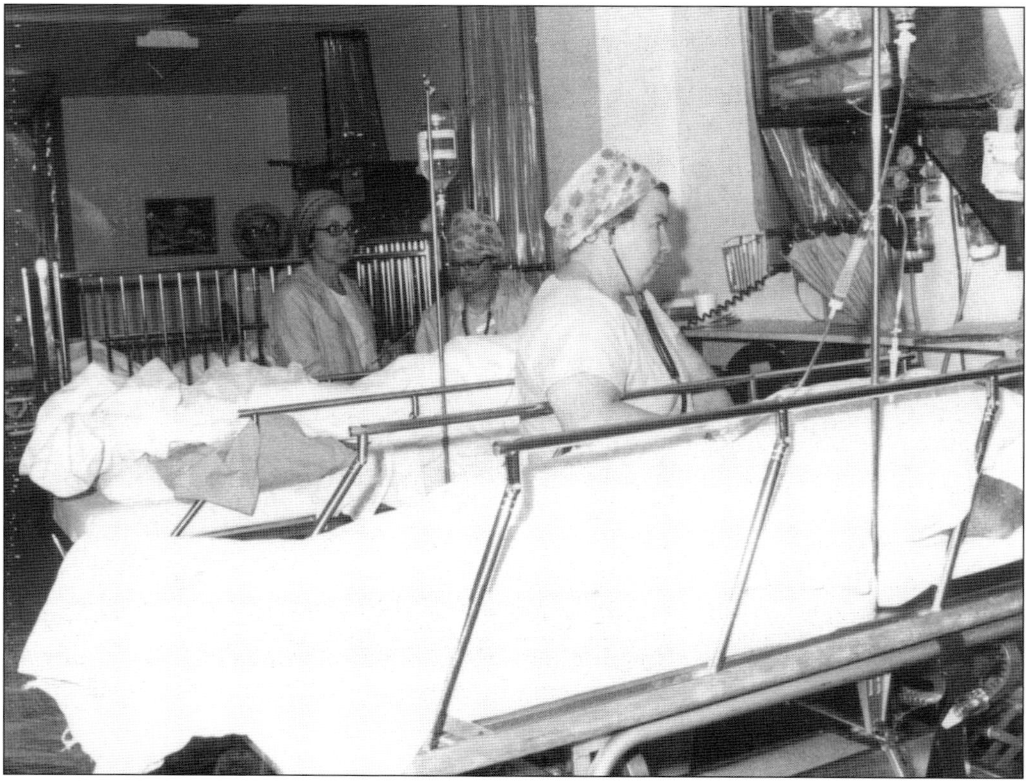

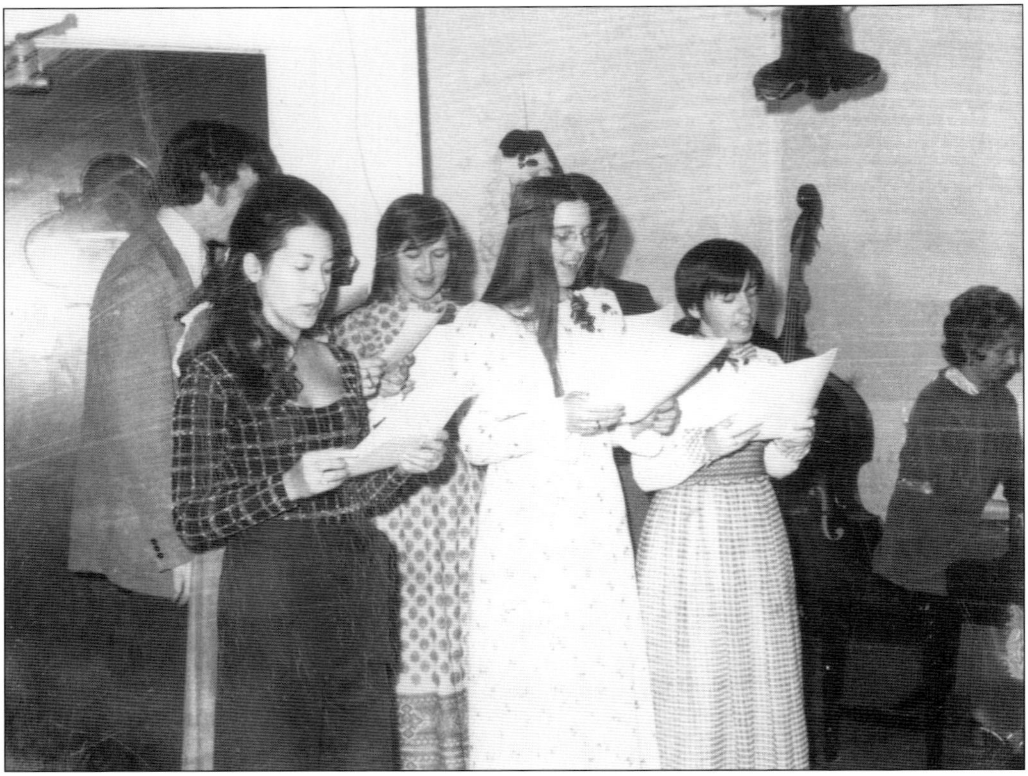

This is the 1972 Franklin County Public Hospital Christmas Party. Employees are singing carols, accompanied by a band. Lynda Zukowski (center, in patterned dress) was a radiology technician then. Today she is director of clinical services, which includes diagnostic imaging.

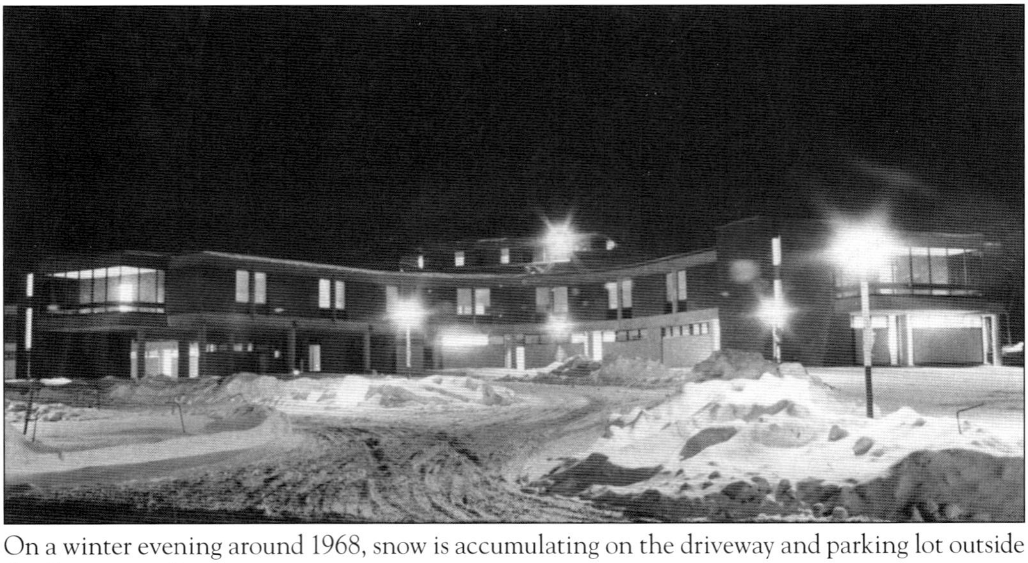

On a winter evening around 1968, snow is accumulating on the driveway and parking lot outside the Emergency Room entrance.

Eight

From FCPH to FMC to BFMC

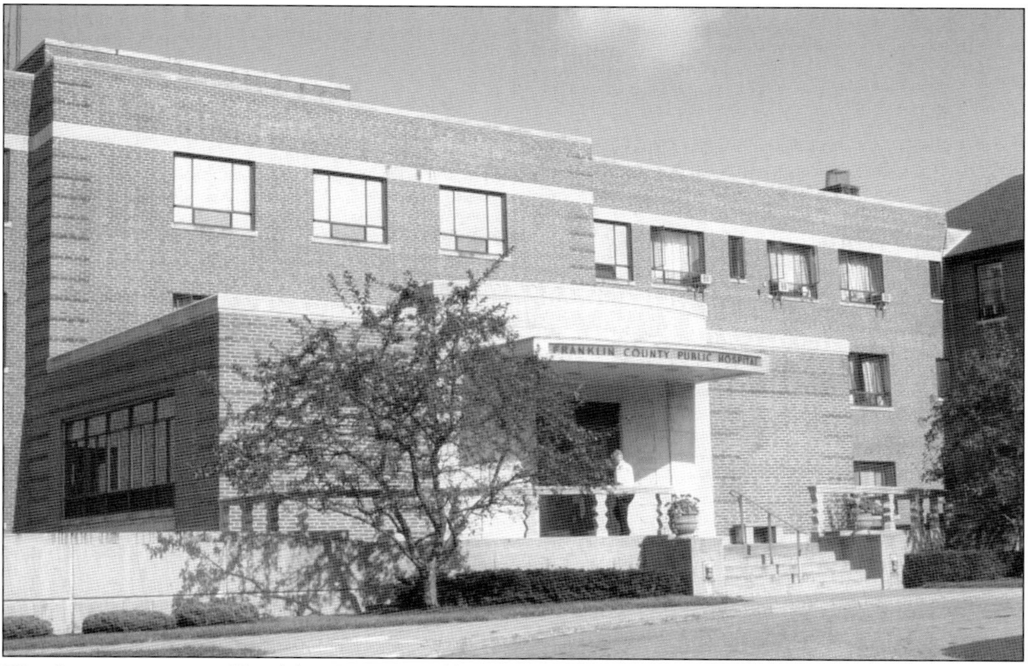

The front entrance to Franklin County Public Hospital is pictured here around 1975. This entrance was replaced by today's covered carport in 1991.

TABLET

FRANKLIN COUNTY PUBLIC HOSPITAL

PUBLISHED BY THE FCPH PUBLIC RELATIONS OFFICE • GREENFIELD, MASS.

January - 1973 Vol. 4 No. 1

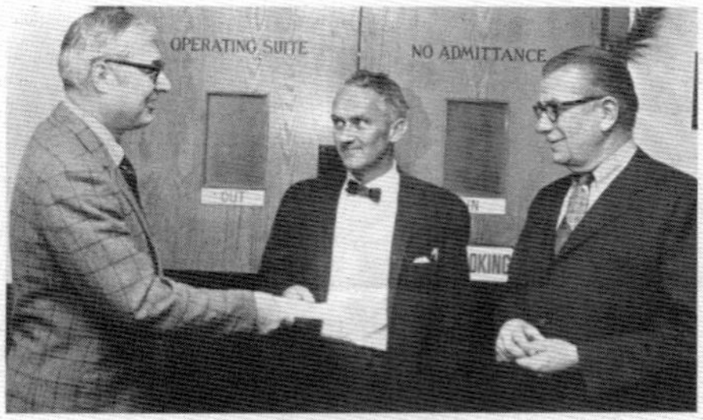

Robert Sawyer, Dr. McClelland, Walker Hosmer

FIRST PLEDGE OF 10,000 DOLLARS TO NEW SURGERY FUND

The Franklin County Association of Insurance Agents, Inc., are the first to make a pledge to the new Surgery Building Fund at the Franklin County Public Hospital.

Mr. Robert Sawyer, representing the Association, presented the first contribution of $3,334 to Mr. Walker Hosmer, President of the Board of Directors and Dr. William K. McClelland, President of the Medical Staff.

The total pledge of $10,000 will be made in three annual payments. Mr. William Christenson, in his acknowledgement of the gift, thanked the Association for its past support of the hospital as well as for the present.

The new proposed addition will provide full surgical facilities on the top floor of a two-story addition and the first floor will be devoted to service and support space. This addition will fill space between two existing buildings and border on Beacon Street.

The surgery will be designed in such a way to maximize patient safety and minimize the risk of infection. Designed to accommodate "day surgery", it is a new concept which will permit a patient having minor surgery to come in the morning and leave at night; avoiding the added cost of hospitalization.

The new surgery fund drive is being planned for the early part of this year. The Franklin County Association of Insurance Agents was organized in 1883. It is a non-profit organization dedicated to improvement of the professional standards of insurance agents doing business in Franklin County. The Association has placed insurance for the hospital for more than 25 years and the members of the Association have been staunch supporters of the hospital, having contributed substantial sums to each of the last two major improvement programs as well as making annual contributions. Mr. Sawyer has been chairman of the Insurance Committee for 14 years.

In 1973, the FCPH board of directors gave approval for a $3-million addition to house new surgery, service, support, and mechanical areas. This photograph from the 1973 FCPH *Tablet* shows Robert Sawyer (of the Franklin County Association of Insurance Agents, the first group to pledge $10,000 to the project) along with Dr. William McClelland, president of the medical staff, and Walker Hosmer, president of the board of directors.

Ground-breaking for the new surgical building was held on July 31, 1974. From left to right are Mr. Hosmer, Joseph Ballard, Dr. William McClelland, Robert Huntress, Robert Mahar, Dr. Robert Speth, Mrs. Aaron Newton, Louise Sessler, Janet Russell, and Carol Haskell. The new building was to be named the Russell Building in recognition of the many contributions to the hospital by Janet Russell and her father, the late William D. Russell.

TABLET

FRANKLIN COUNTY PUBLIC HOSPITAL

PUBLISHED BY THE FCPH PUBLIC RELATIONS OFFICE • GREENFIELD, MASS.

August – Vol. 5 – No. 7

GROUNDBREAKING

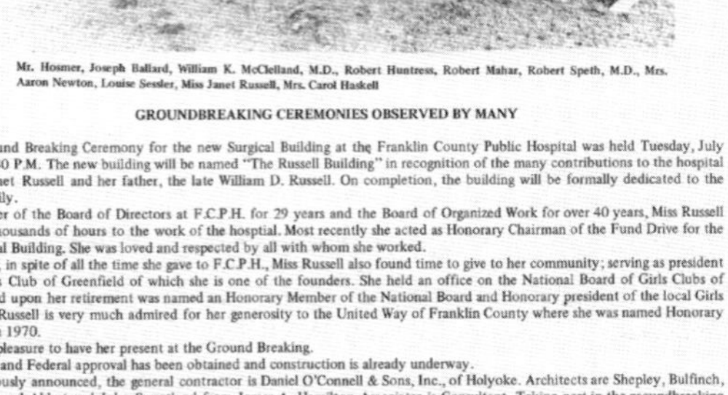

Mr. Hosmer, Joseph Ballard, William K. McClelland, M.D., Robert Huntress, Robert Mahar, Robert Speth, M.D., Mrs. Aaron Newton, Louise Sessler, Miss Janet Russell, Mrs. Carol Haskell

GROUNDBREAKING CEREMONIES OBSERVED BY MANY

The Ground Breaking Ceremony for the new Surgical Building at the Franklin County Public Hospital was held Tuesday, July 31st, at 1:30 P.M. The new building will be named "The Russell Building" in recognition of the many contributions to the hospital by Miss Janet Russell and her father, the late William D. Russell. On completion, the building will be formally dedicated to the Russell family.

A member of the Board of Directors at F.C.P.H. for 29 years and the Board of Organized Work for over 40 years, Miss Russell has given thousands of hours to the work of the hosptial. Most recently she acted as Honorary Chairman of the Fund Drive for the New Surgical Building. She was loved and respected by all with whom she worked.

However, in spite of all the time she gave to F.C.P.H., Miss Russell also found time to give to her community; serving as president of the Girls Club of Greenfield of which she is one of the founders. She held an office on the National Board of Girls Clubs of America and upon her retirement was named an Honorary Member of the National Board and Honorary president of the local Girls Club. Miss Russell is very much admired for her generosity to the United Way of Franklin County where she was named Honorary Chairman in 1970.

It was a pleasure to have her present at the Ground Breaking.

All State and Federal approval has been obtained and construction is already underway.

As previously announced, the general contractor is Daniel O'Connell & Sons, Inc., of Holyoke. Architects are Shepley, Bulfinch, Richardson and Abbot and John Sweetland from James A. Hamilton Associates is Consultant. Taking part in the groundbreaking ceremonies were: William Christenson, Mr. Walker Hosmer, Robert Speth, M.D., William K. McClelland, M.D., Mrs. Carol Haskell, Miss Louise Sessler, Mr. Joseph Ballard, Robert Huntress, Robert Mahar, Mrs. Aaron Newton and our Guest of Honor, Miss Janet Russell. Noticeably absent was Mr. Howard Cadwell, General Chairman of the Fund Drive. Mr. Cadwell is vacationing after the hectic activities of the Fund Raising Campaign which at the present time stands at $856,000.00. His "resting" vacation was spent "back-packing" through the Rockies.

Dr. William McClelland was a long-time surgeon at FCPH/BFMC and had a general surgery practice in Greenfield for 35 years, retiring in 1991. He was president of the BFMC medical staff from 1972 to 1974. A classical musician, Dr. McClelland played flute, and later bassoon, with the Pioneer Valley Symphony Orchestra, and was occasionally seen strolling around the hospital with a bassoon reed in his mouth. His son, Dr. Alan McClelland, also a surgeon and current BFMC physician, was president of the medical staff from January 2009 to December 2012.

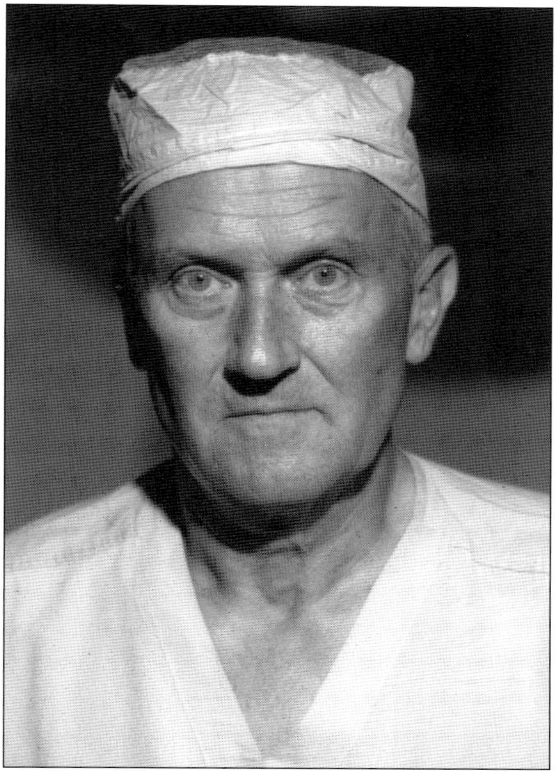

Allen Abercrombie and Janet Russell of the BOOW chart an interim fundraising total of $786,629 in August 1974. Procedures would fund the $3-million Russell Building.

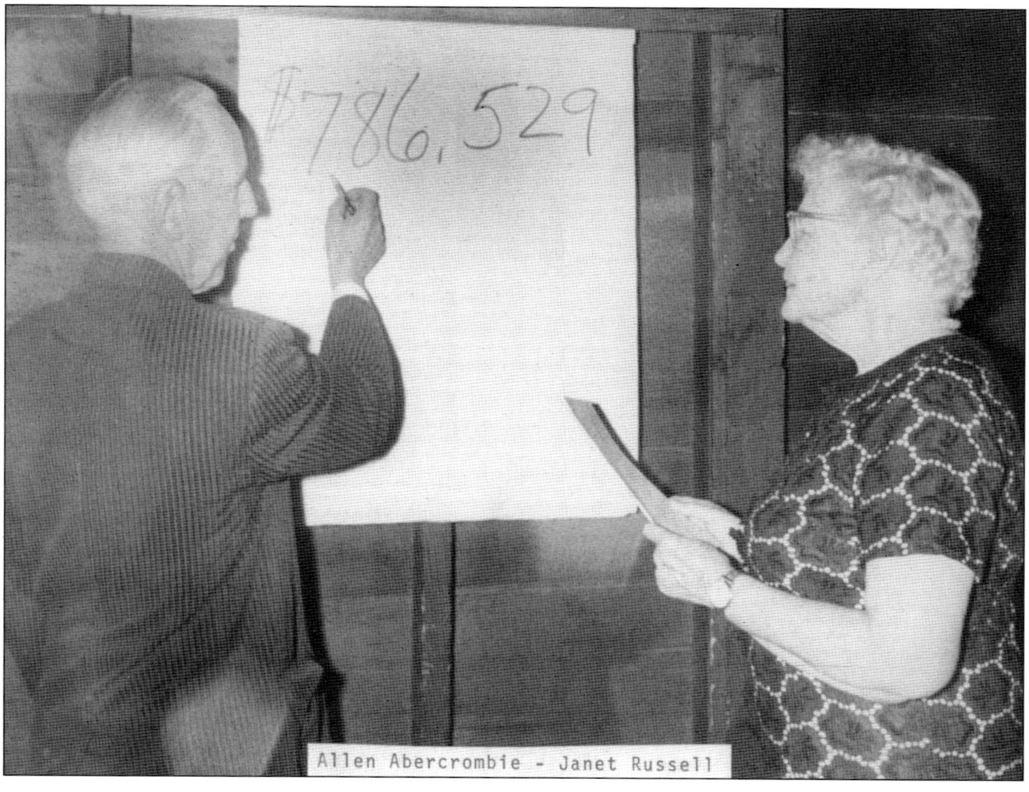

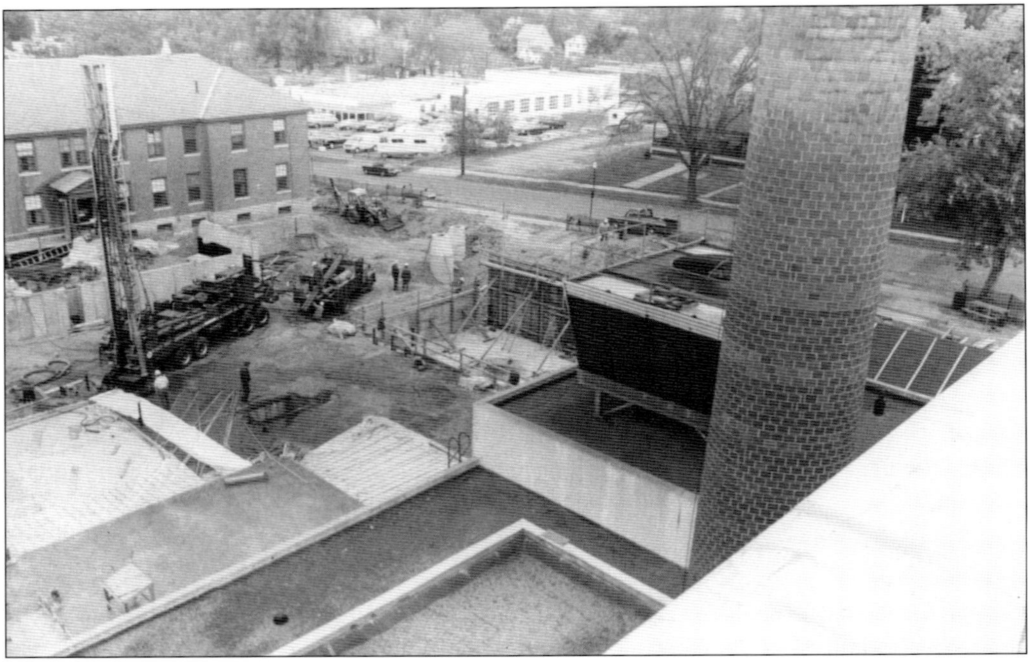

This view from the roof of the main hospital shows the excavation and foundations for the new Russell Building. The building to the left is the former FCPH School of Nursing, now repurposed as a medical office building. Across Beacon Street, the parking lot at Brown's Motors is full of vehicles.

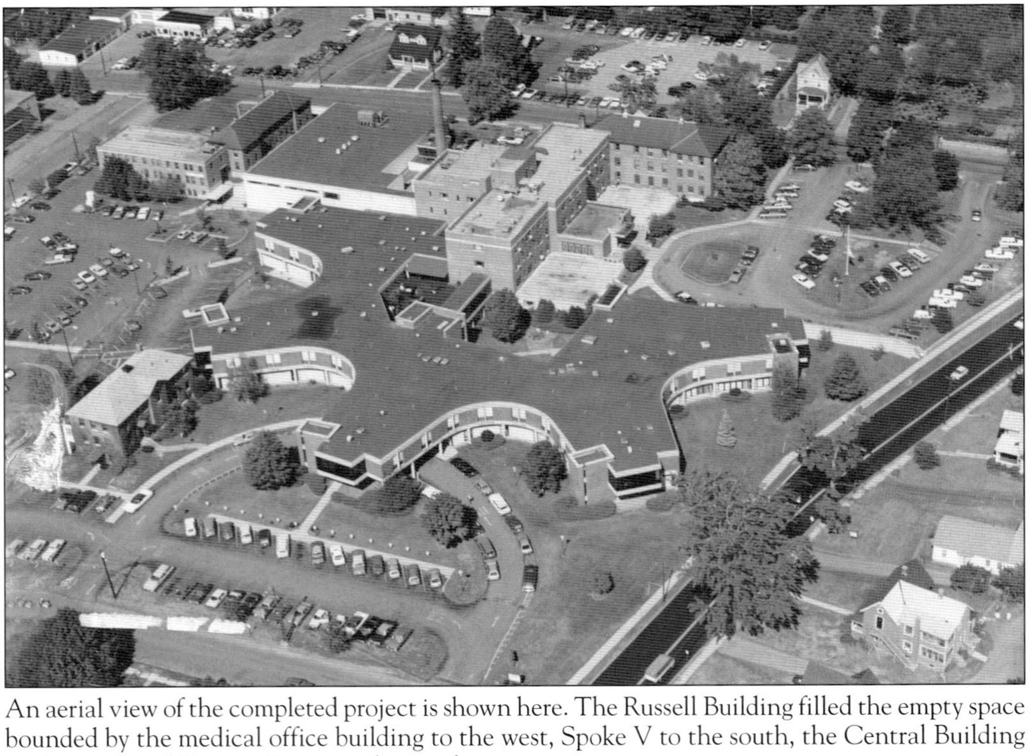

An aerial view of the completed project is shown here. The Russell Building filled the empty space bounded by the medical office building to the west, Spoke V to the south, the Central Building to the east, and Beacon Street to the north.

This is a formal photograph of William D. Russell. The 1975 expansion project was named the Russell Building in recognition of the many contributions to the hospital by William D. Russell and his daughter, Janet Russell. Janet Russell was a member of the board of directors of Franklin County Public Hospital for 29 years and a member of the BOOW for over 40 years.

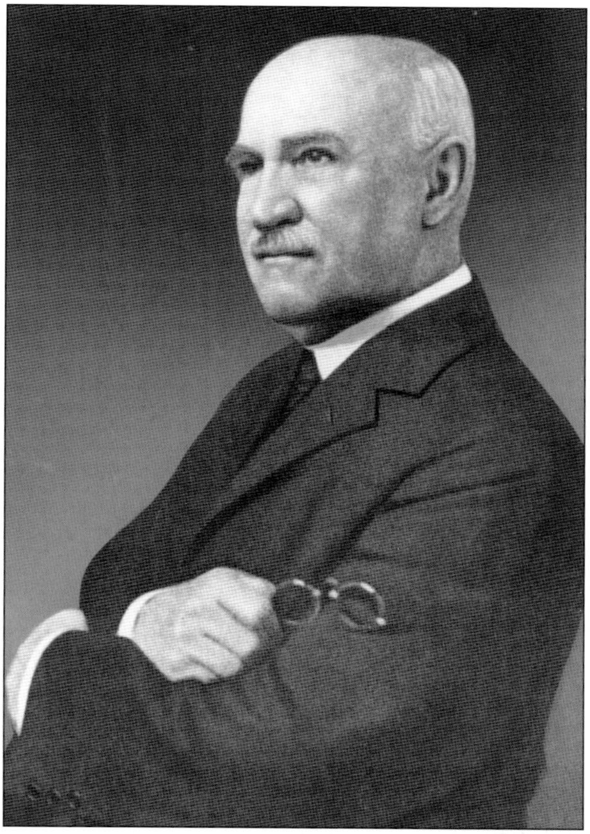

The open house and ribbon-cutting for the new surgery wing was held on February 9, 1975. The speaker is Burt Winer, chairman of the board of directors of FCPH. To his right are Bill Zwemke, assistant director; Walker Hosmer, past president of the board of directors; and Janet Russell.

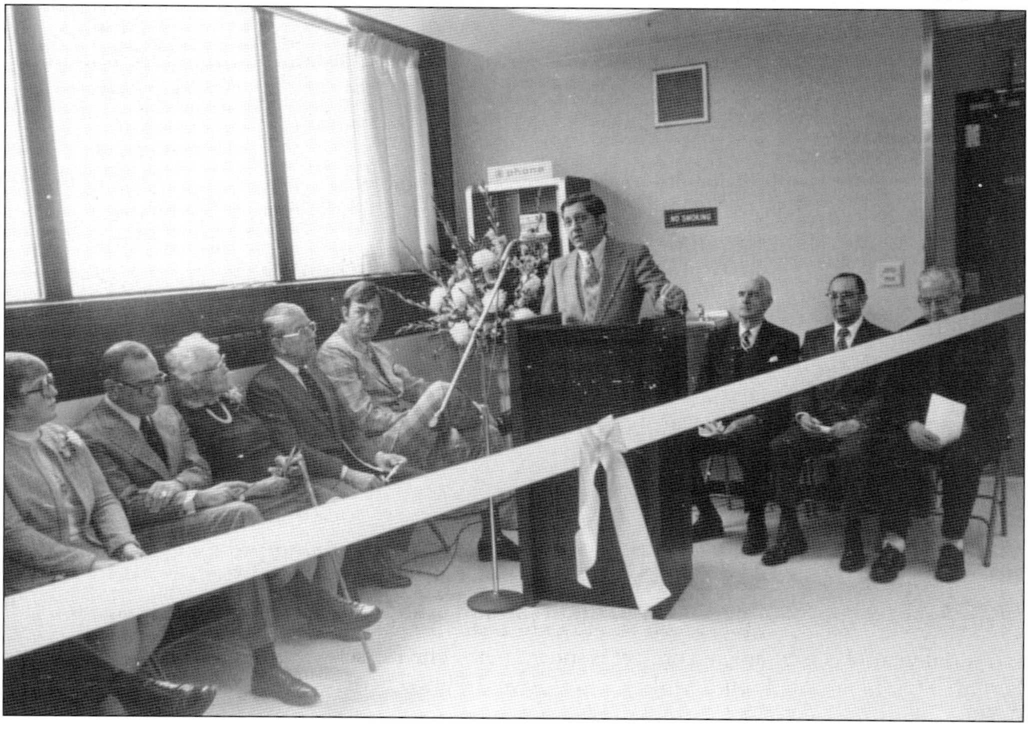

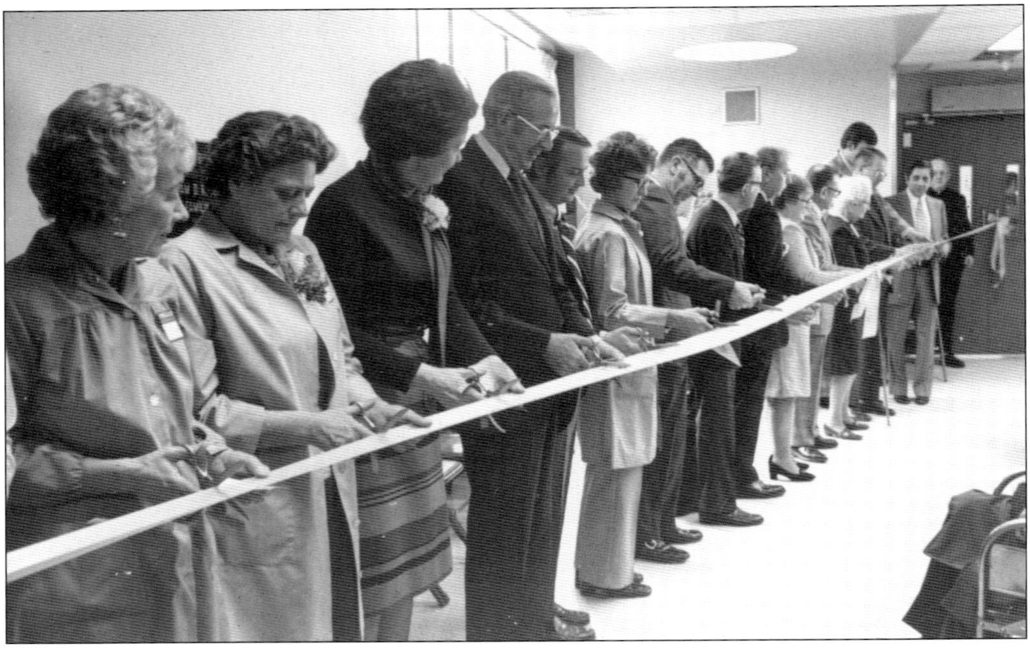

Members of the Board of Organized Work and various guests participate in the ribbon-cutting ceremony on February 9, 1975.

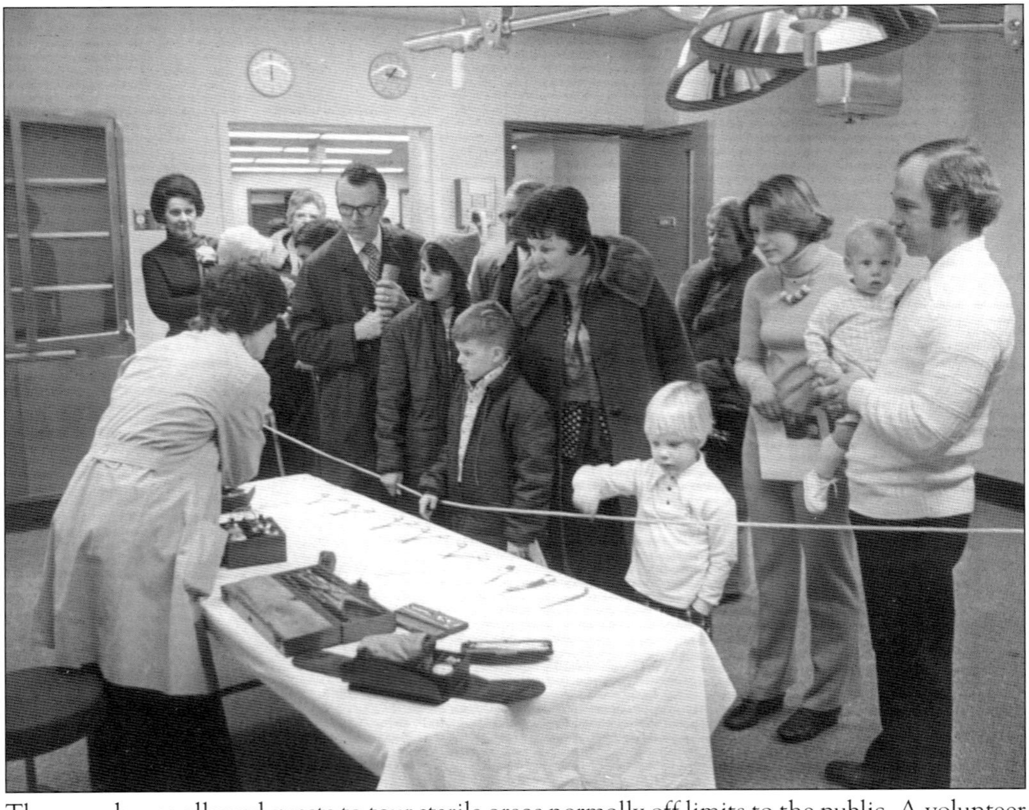

The open house allowed guests to tour sterile areas normally off limits to the public. A volunteer displays vintage and modern surgical instruments inside one of the new operating rooms.

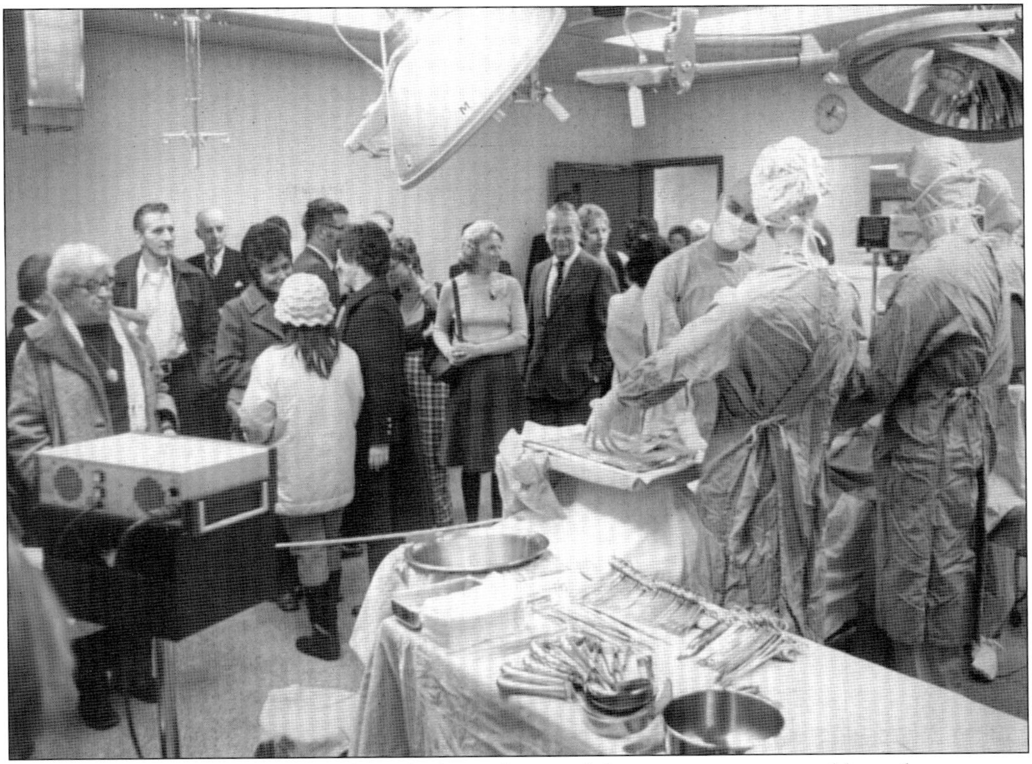

Nurses fully gowned, gloved, and masked stand around the operating room table to demonstrate their normal daily routine to the open house audience.

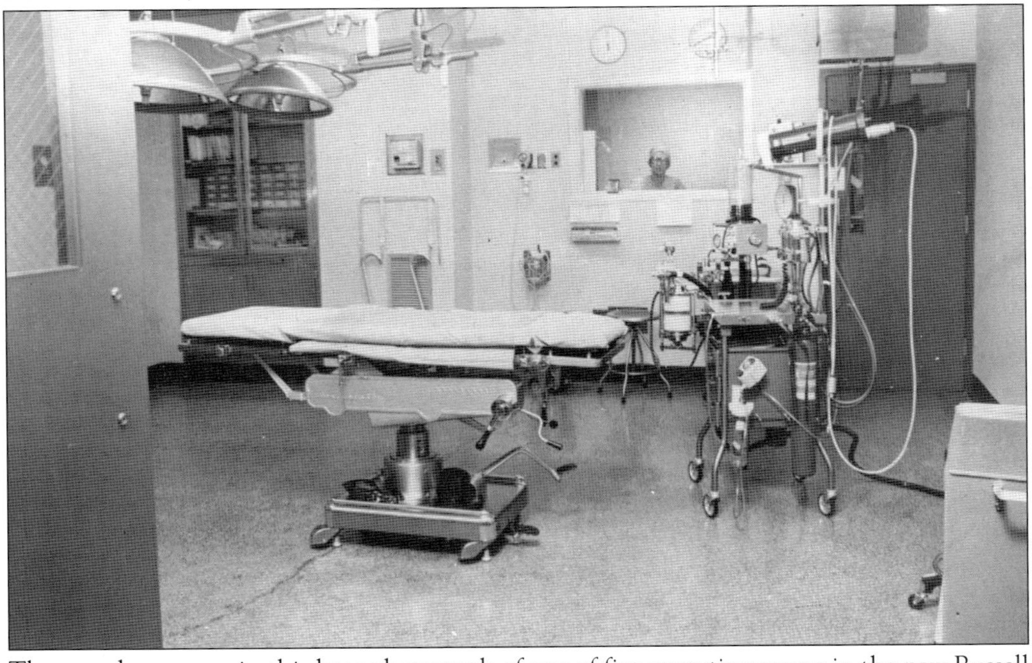

The crowds are gone in this later photograph of one of five operating rooms in the new Russell Building. The observation window allows surgeons and nurses to watch preparation of the patient while they are scrubbing at the sink.

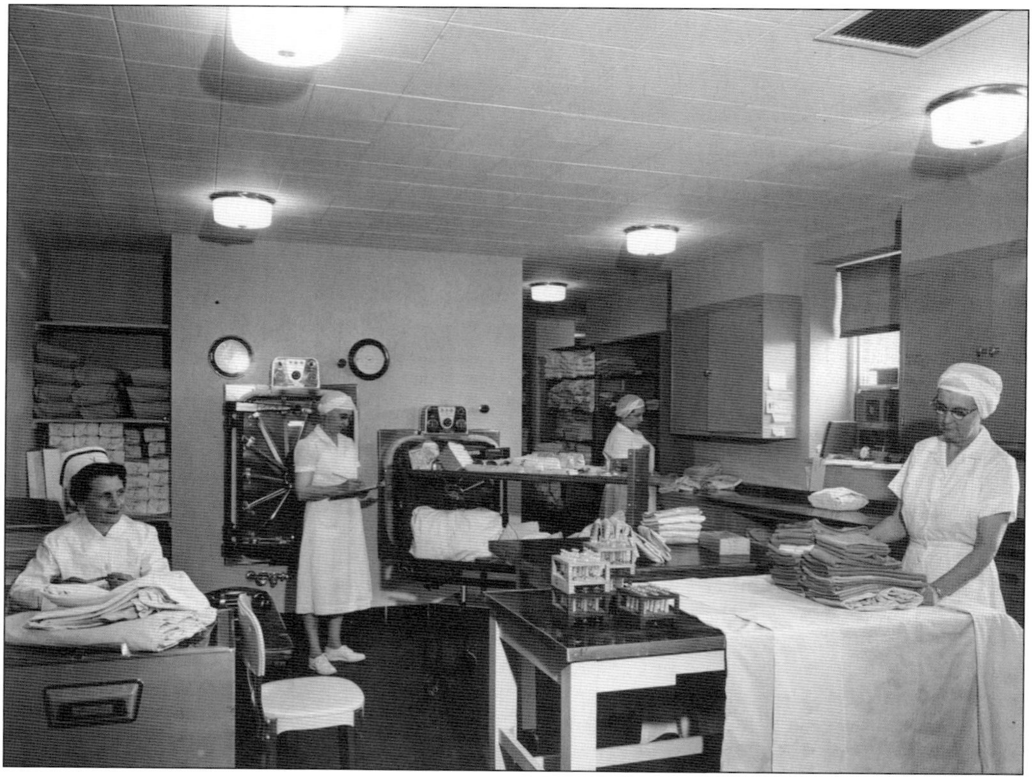

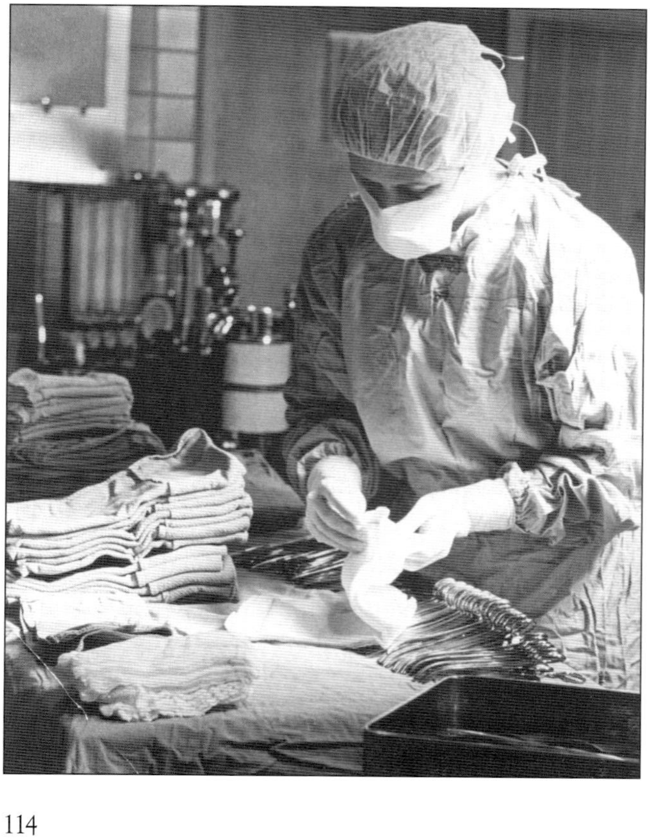

The Sterile Processing Department (SPD) is an essential but often invisible service provided by hospitals. Here, surgical drapes and instruments are sorted, cleaned, sterilized, and then packed for reuse. The Russell Building incorporated new SPD facilities, replacing outmoded equipment in the Central Building. The 1975 Russell Building SPD will soon be supplanted by the 2016 surgical building currently under construction.

A scrub nurse in the operating room prepares gauze sponges, towels, and surgical instruments. In 1975, FCPH logged 40,710 patient days and 5,526 admissions and had an average daily census (ADC) of 149 patients. Today, with more outpatient procedures and shorter lengths-of-stay, ADC rarely exceeds 90.

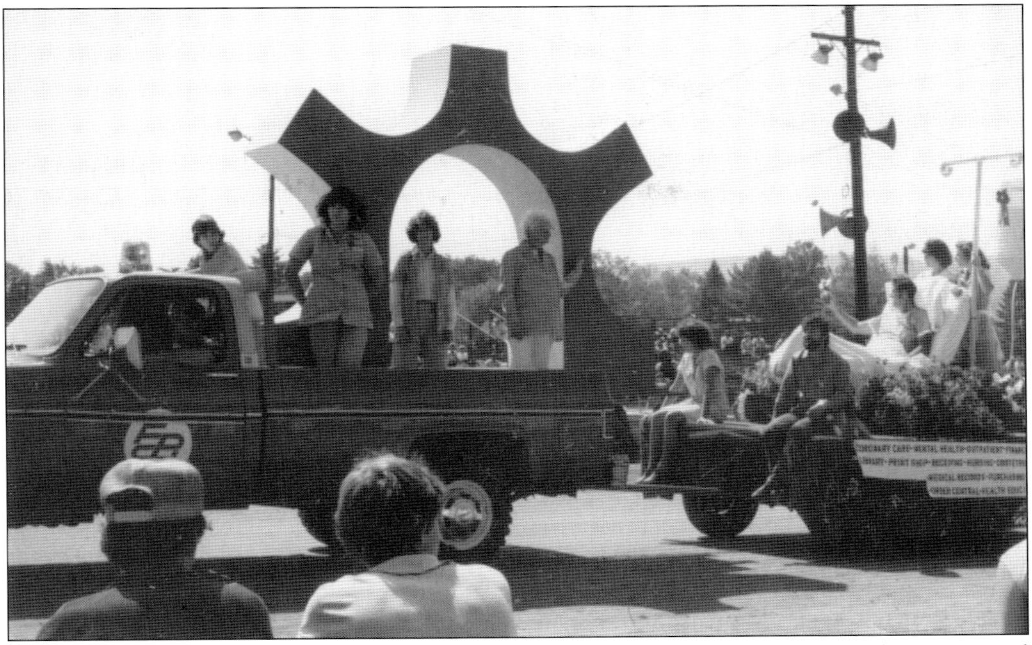

The unique and award-winning design of the Spokes was incorporated into the hospital's promotional materials. In this photograph from the summer of 1981, a truck with an older FCPH logo tows a float carrying a representation of the Spokes in the opening parade for the Franklin County Fair.

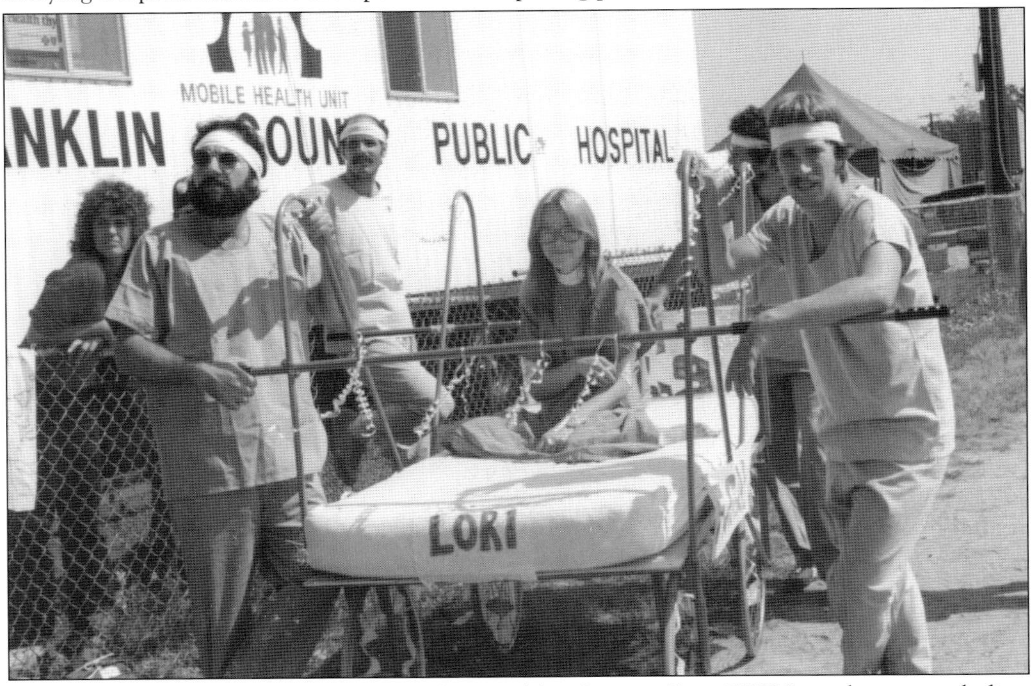

The bed race was an annual event at the Franklin County Fair. FCPH employees, including Bob Perlman (with beard); Lori Canedy Tyler, RN, seated on the bed; and Jim Bassett (far right) get ready for the race. FCPH's mobile health unit is in the background. The logo shown on the mobile unit, depicting two adults and two children, would eventually be incorporated into the logo for Baystate Health.

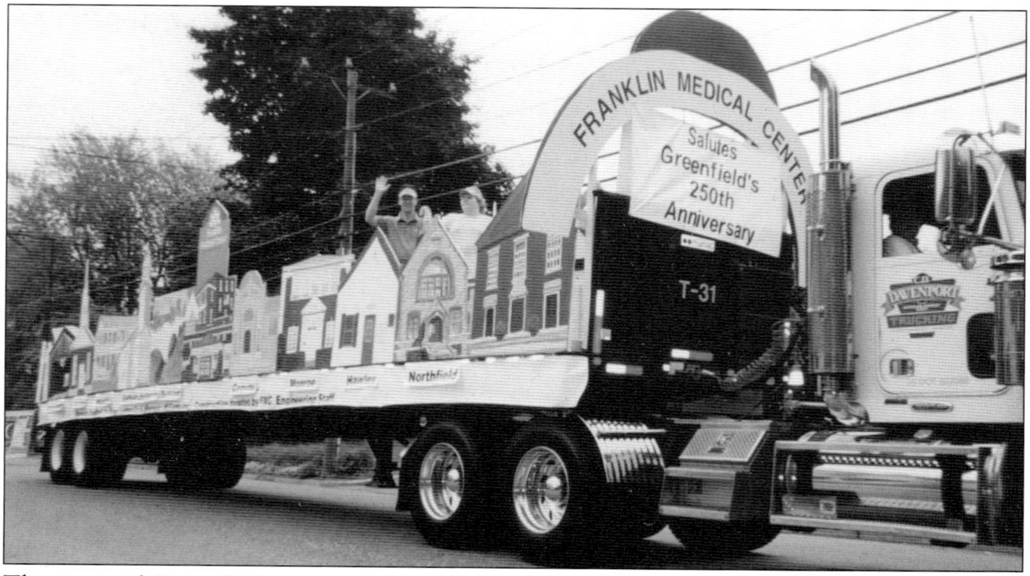
FRANKLIN MEDICAL CENTER
Salutes
Greenfield's
250th
Anniversary
T-31
Northfield
The town of Greenfield was settled in 1686 and founded in 1753. In 2003, Franklin Medical Center engineering constructed a float with historic buildings celebrating Greenfield's 250th anniversary.

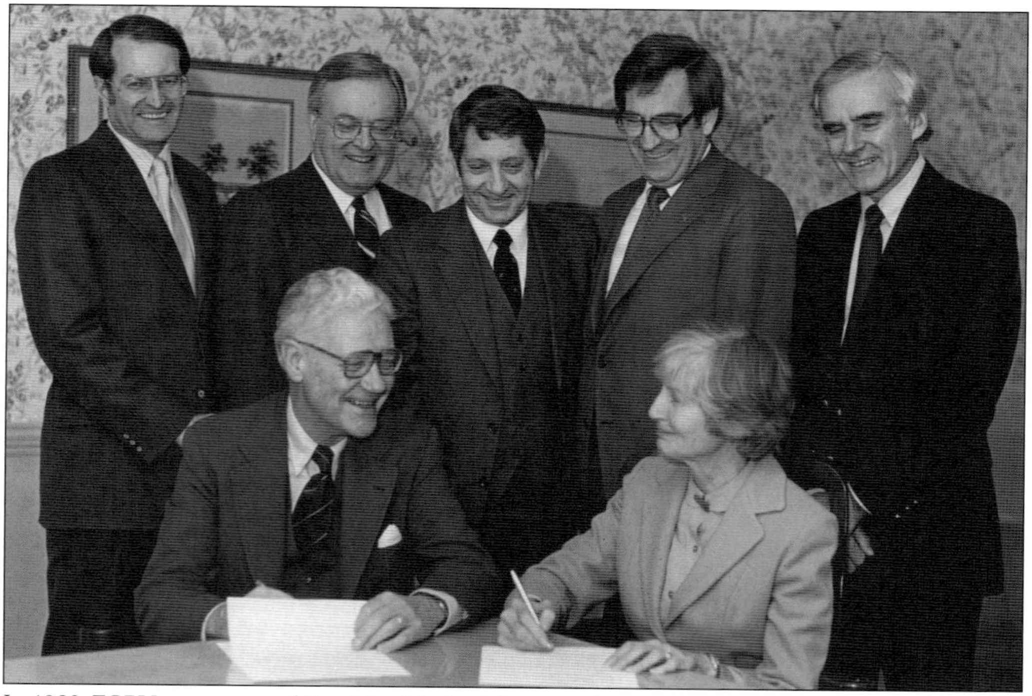
In 1983, FCPH was renamed Franklin Medical Center. That same year, FMC signed a cooperation agreement with Baystate Medical Center in Springfield, Massachusetts, planning to share clinical, lab, library, and medical education resources. By 1986, FMC and BMC merged to form Baystate Health Systems (BHS), with 3,822 total employees and an $87-million payroll. At the ceremony creating BHS, Herbert Almgren from BMC sits next to Jeanne B. Smith, chairwoman of the FMC board of directors. In the back row are Dr. Max Cloud, Harry Gifford (president of BMC), Burton Winer, Eugene E. Loubier (president of FMC), and Dr. Eugene Whittier.

Harlan Smith was president of Franklin Medical Center from 1987 to 2000. During his tenure, a $5.7-million expansion and renovation construction project was undertaken that included the new addition to the front of the building. BFMC also celebrated its 100th anniversary in 1995.

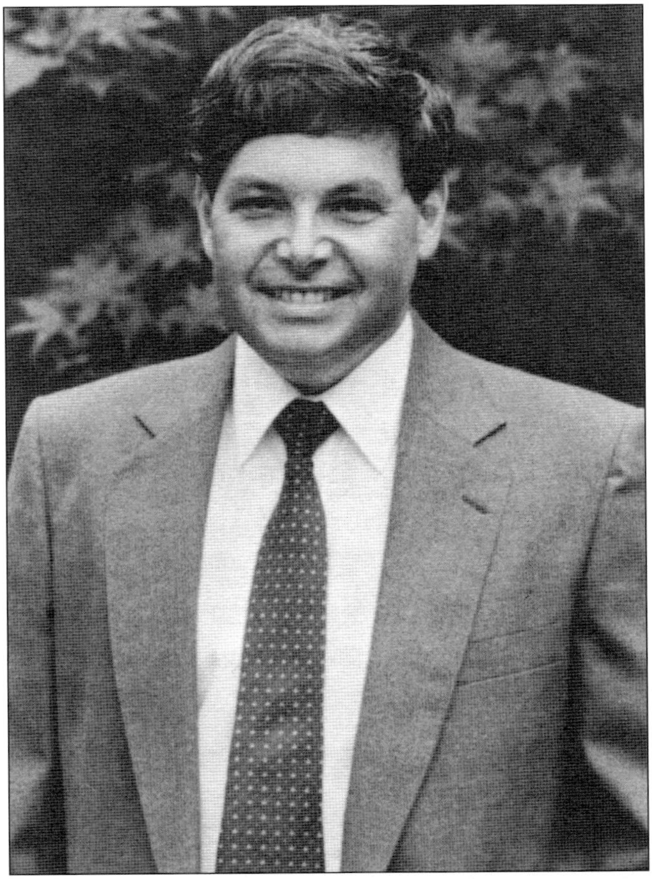

Radiologist Howard "Howie" Natenshon, also known as "Dr. Nate," joined FCPH in 1975 and continues to practice today, celebrating his 40-year anniversary in 2015. He has a special interest in cancer treatment and was instrumental in creating the annual fundraiser Wheeling for Healing with Bruce Mainville, nuclear med technician, in which proceeds from the cycling event are used for cancer patients at BFMC.

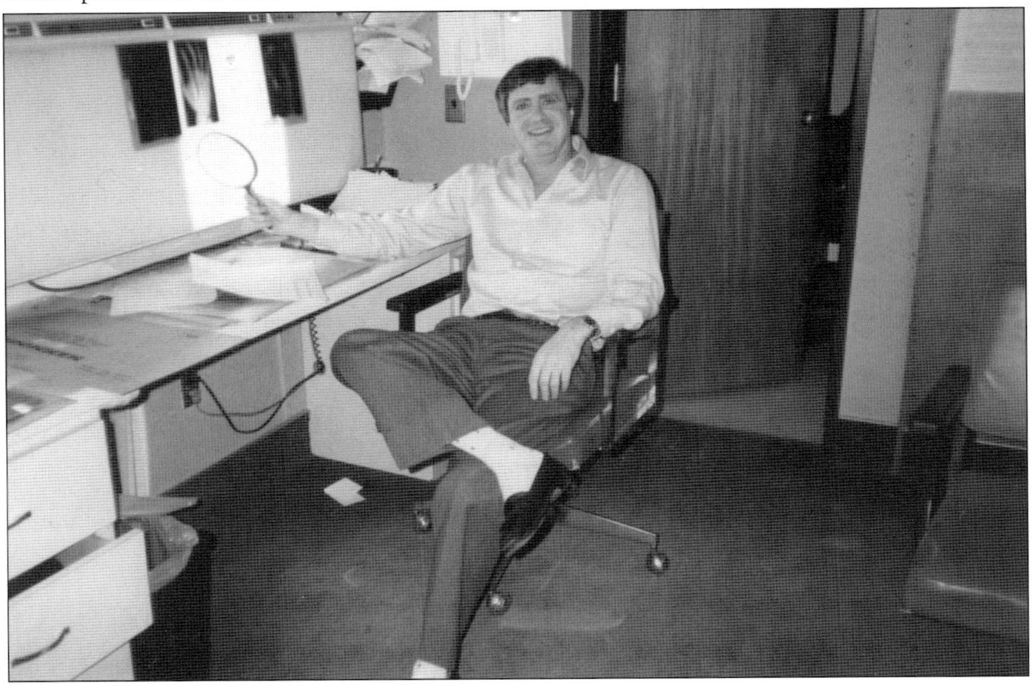

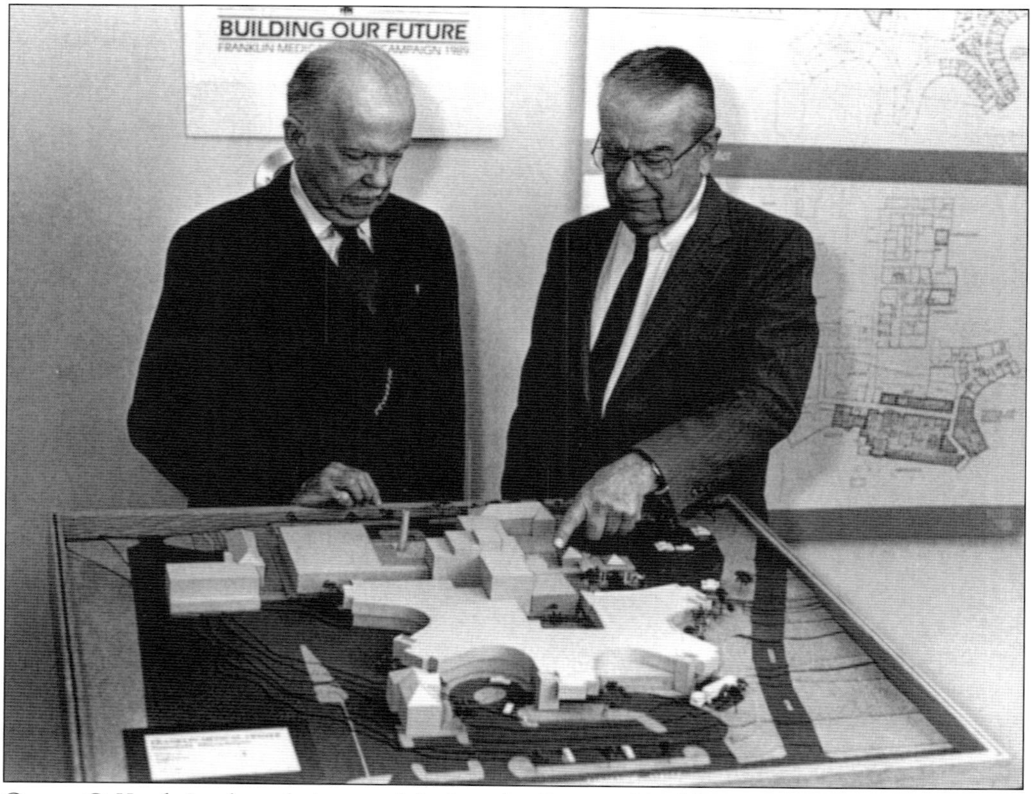

George C. Keady Jr., then chairman of the board at Baystate Health Systems, and Walker Hosmer, honorary chairman of the capital fund drive, examine an architect's model. In 1989, a capital campaign was announced with a goal of $1.2 million in fundraising to support a $5.7-million expansion of the hospital. The campaign raised $2.17 million, exceeding the goal. (Photograph by Paul Franz, GR.)

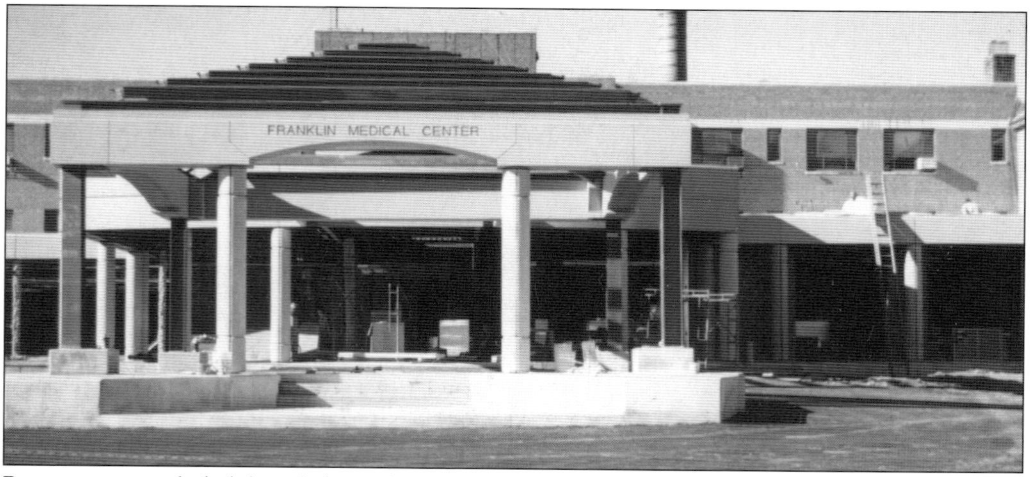

Renovations included demolishing the Central Building entrance and eventually expanding the lobby to High Street. New space would be created for physical therapy, a department that grew from just over 2,000 visits in 1969 to nearly 15,000 in 1988. The project would also consolidate kidney dialysis, cancer treatment, admitting, endoscopy, and preadmission testing into more convenient, larger, and renovated quarters.

Nine

BFMC IN THE 21ST CENTURY

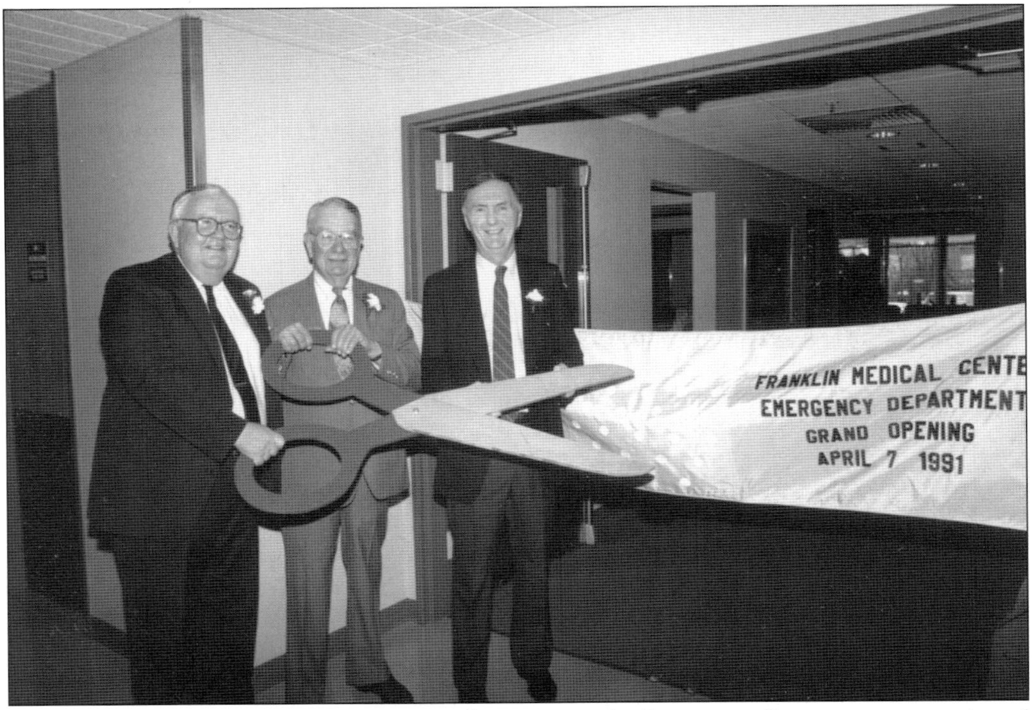

Steady growth in the volume of patients seeking care in the Emergency Department necessitated a complete redesign and expansion beyond its original confines on the ground floor of Spoke III. The newly enlarged facility was dedicated on April 7, 1991. Shown at the ribbon-cutting are, from left to right, David Curry, who was board chairman in 1995–1996; Walker Hosmer, honorary life trustee; and Peter Elliott, member of the executive committee of the board of trustees.

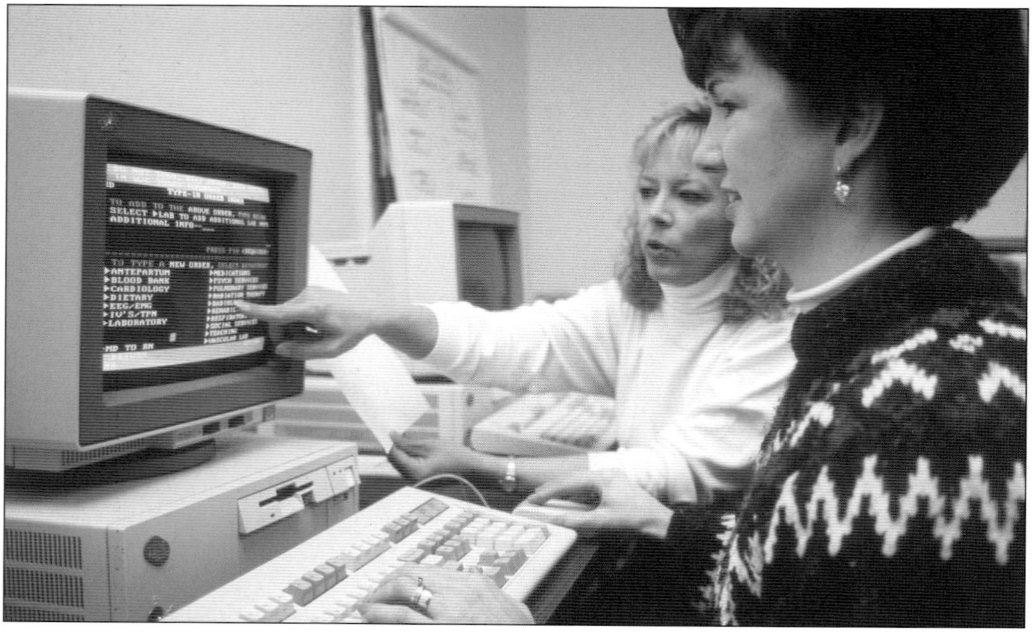

Baystate Health was an early adopter of electronic medical records in the early 1990s. The Patient Care Information System (PCIS) was relatively primitive by today's standards but allowed electronic ordering with built-in safeguards to improve medication safety. Here, Jan Peterson (left) demonstrates how to insert orders for radiation therapy with Gail Shattuck, RN (right).

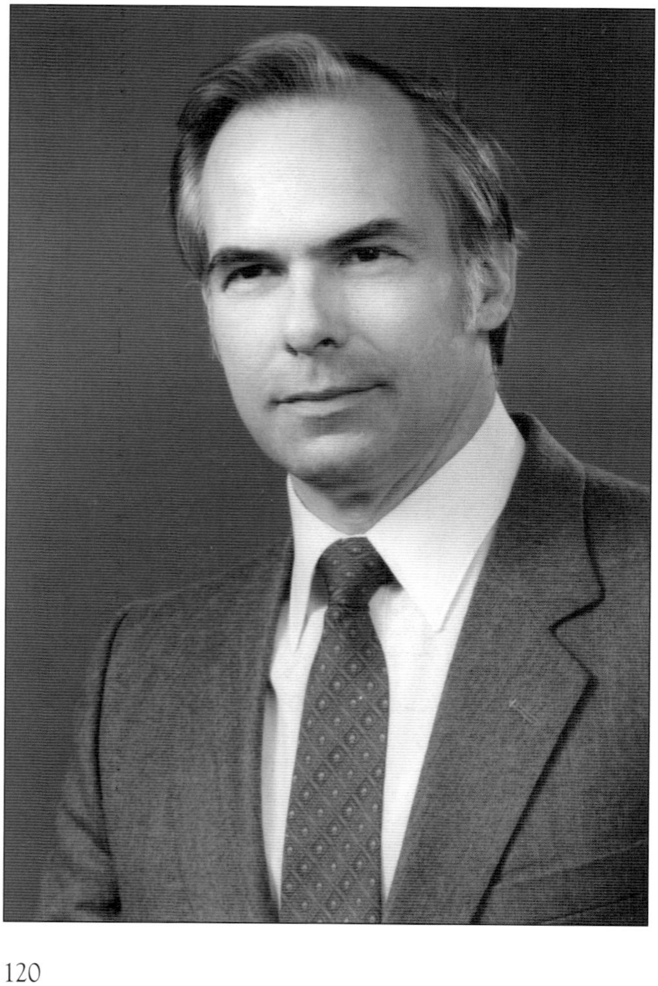

Dr. William E. Callahan is pictured while president of the Massachusetts Medical Society (MMS) in 1992–1993. In his 44-year career as an obstetrician at FCPH/BFMC, he delivered some 5,000 babies. He was a strong supporter of efforts to reduce domestic violence. Dr. Callahan retired from practice in 2015. He is one of four FCPH/BFMC physicians to have headed the MMS.

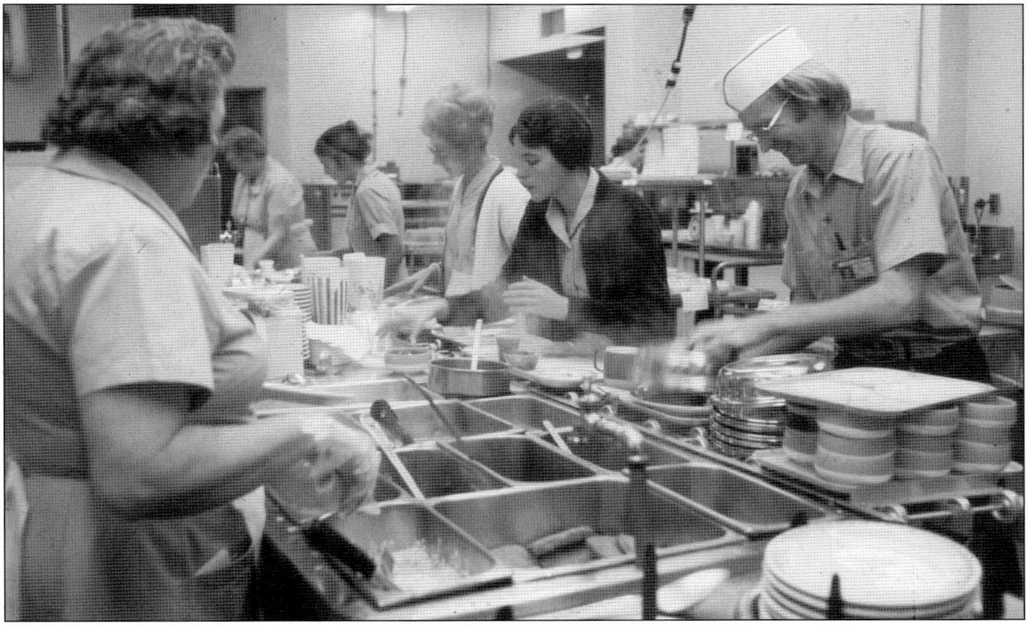

Hospitals are not only temples of healing but must also function as hotels and restaurants. The kitchen crew is pictured assembling patient trays. At far right is Roland Trombley, who began working at FCPH in 1973 and is still an employee in 2016.

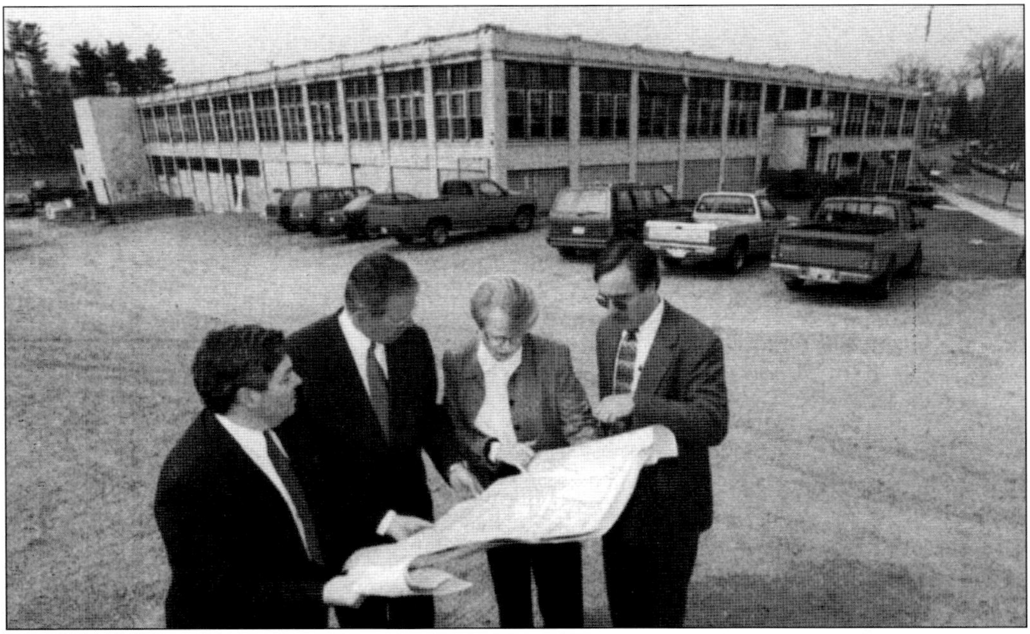

Greenfield Tap & Die, founded in Greenfield in 1872, was once the world's largest manufacturer of machine tools. Other hand tool, machine tool, and cutlery operations once flourished in Franklin County before foreign competition began to take its toll in the 1980s. In July 1993, FMC agreed to purchase the recently vacated office and warehouse building at 48 Sanderson Street. In this photograph from April 1998, Harlan Smith, president of FMC; Michael Daly, president of Baystate Health; Princy Stotz, vice-chair of the Baystate Health board; and Ross Gorman of the Baystate Health board examine plans for an ambulatory care center. (Photograph by Paul Franz, GR.)

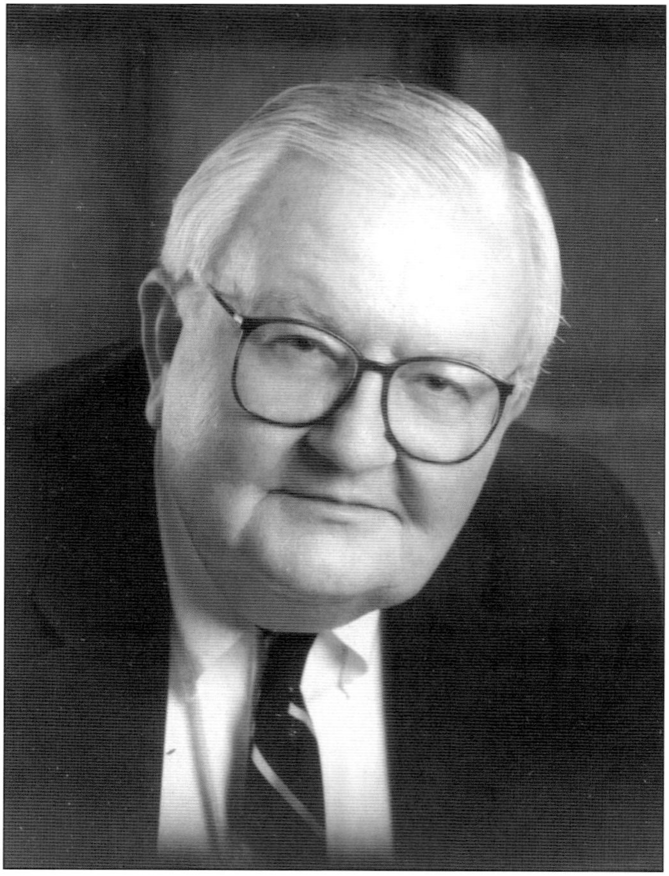

David P. Currey Jr. (1935–2012) was chairman of the board of BFMC in 1995–1996 and on the board of directors of Baystate Health from 1993 to 2000. After a stint in the US Army Center-Intelligence Corps from 1958 to 1961, he entered banking, becoming president of the Bank of New England of Franklin County from 1983 to 1987, followed by other positions in insurance and banking.

Orthopedic surgeon Dr. Jeffrey Hayer is shown educating community members. BFMC has long sponsored Senior Class events to provide local citizens with information on health and wellness.

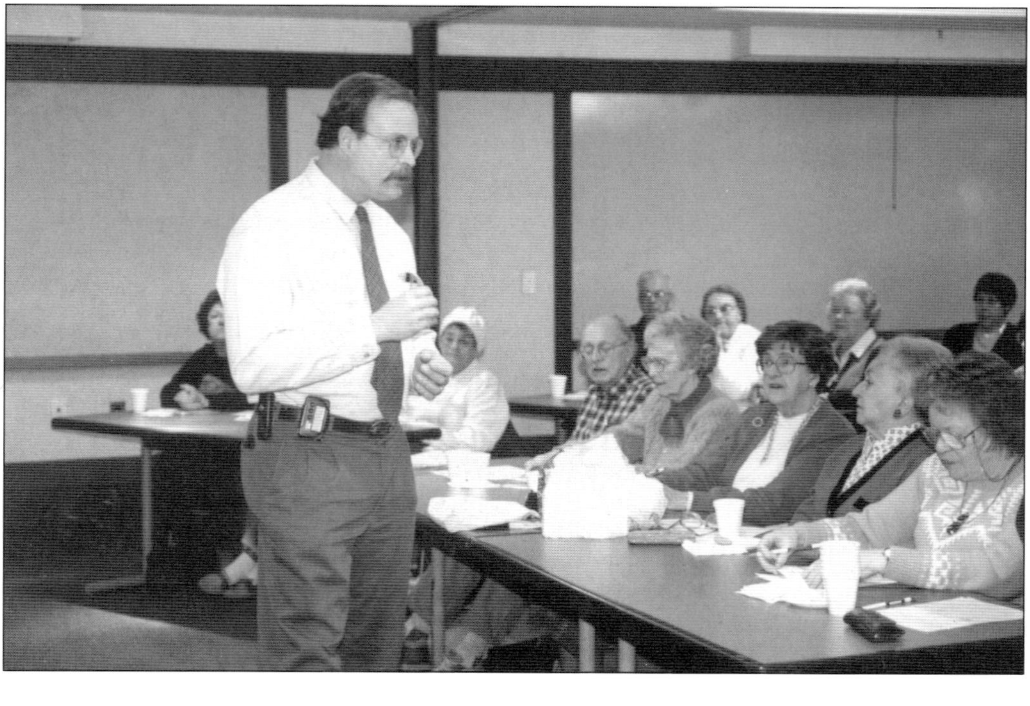

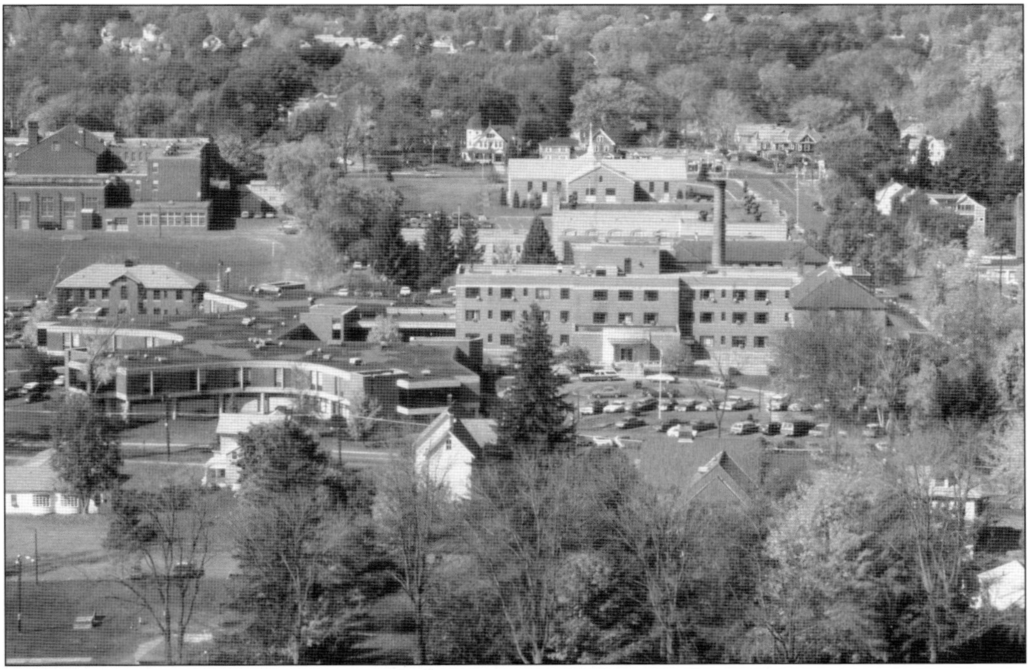

BFMC is on High Street, which parallels the northern Pocumtuck Range. This view from the top of Poet's Seat Tower, taken in the late 1980s, shows the Holy Trinity School and the Blessed Sacrament Church in the distance.

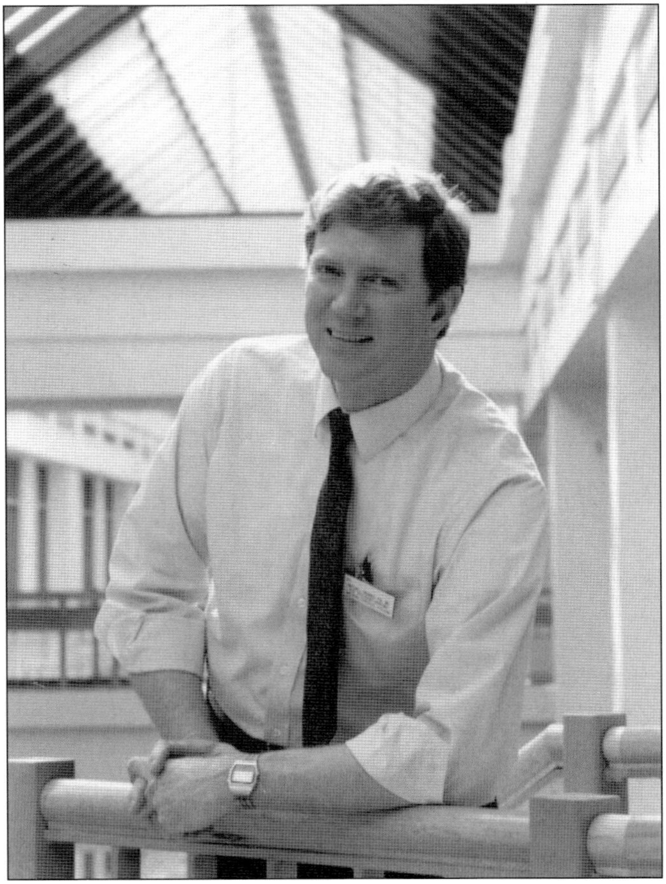

Michael Skinner is pictured in 2006. During his tenure as president of BFMC, the major 2005–2007 renovation and expansion project was launched, supported by a $6-million community campaign. The project expanded the Emergency and Radiology Departments and updated the ICU and Spokes III and IV.

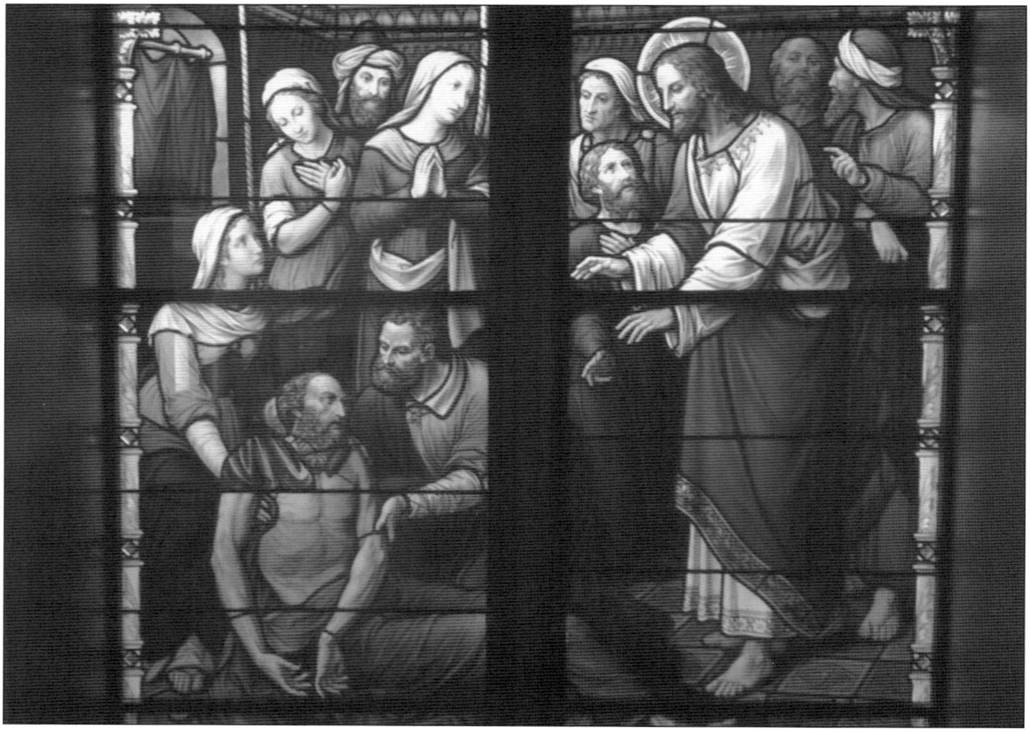

Christ Healing the Paralytic is the title of the stained-glass window incorporated into the BFMC chapel during renovations in the early 1990s. The vintage stained glass was salvaged from a closed church in Holyoke, Massachusetts, through the efforts of Channing L. "Joe" Bete, a long-time supporter of the hospital. (TLH.)

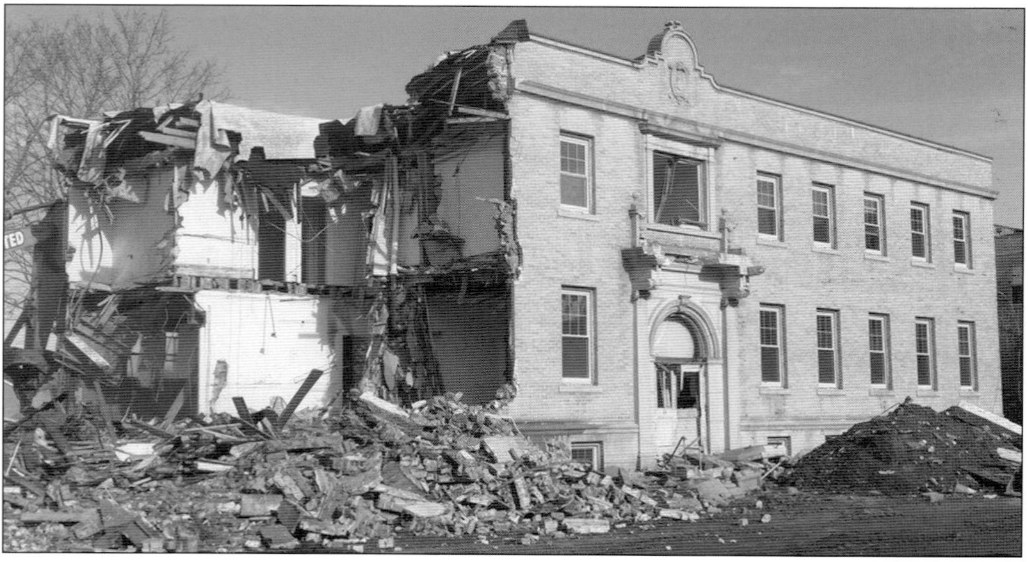

Holy Trinity Parish in Greenfield opened its parochial school in 1929 at the corner of Beacon and North Streets. Despite efforts of parents, alumni, and parishioners, it struggled with low enrollment in its latter years and closed at the end of the 2011 academic year. The building was sold to BFMC, and dismantled in 2015 to provide parking facilities displaced by construction of the new surgical building. (TLH.)

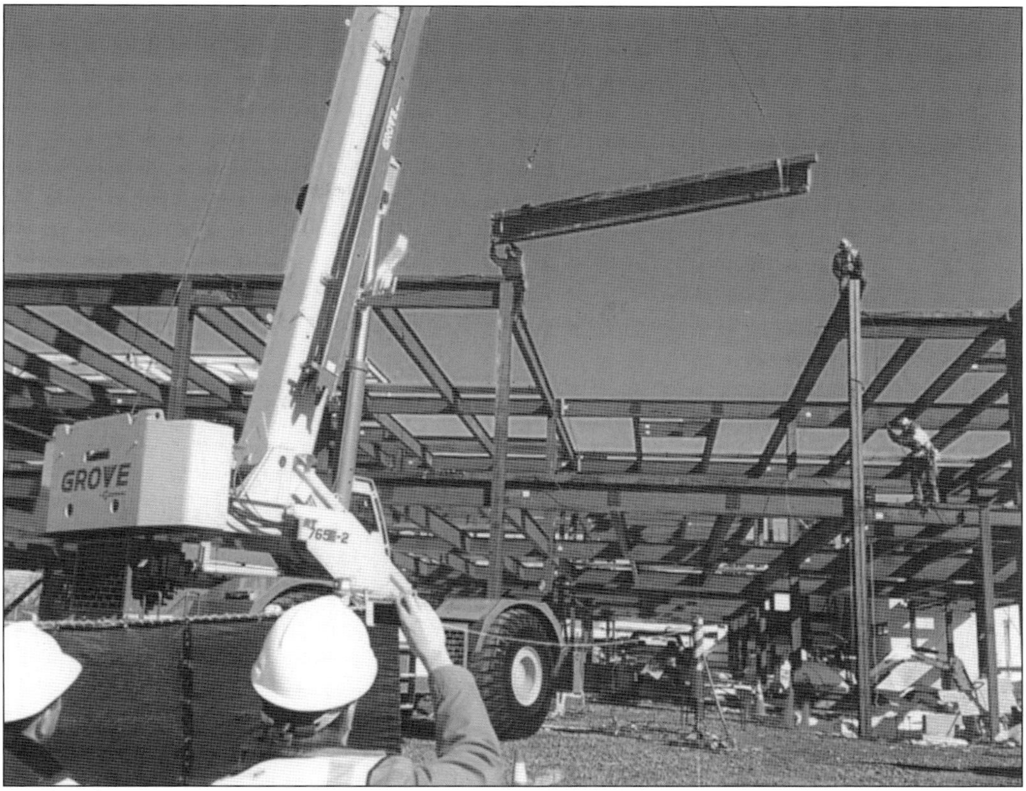

Steelwork is going up for the new surgical building in January 2015. The beam being raised in this photograph was signed by staff and community members. (Photograph by Daren Gray.)

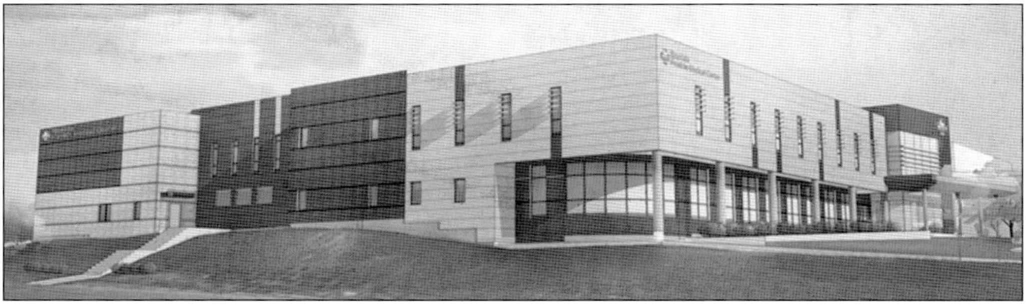
An architect's rendering shows the new surgical building, due to open in 2016. The upper level supports space for four operating rooms, pre-operation care, sterile processing, and other support functions.

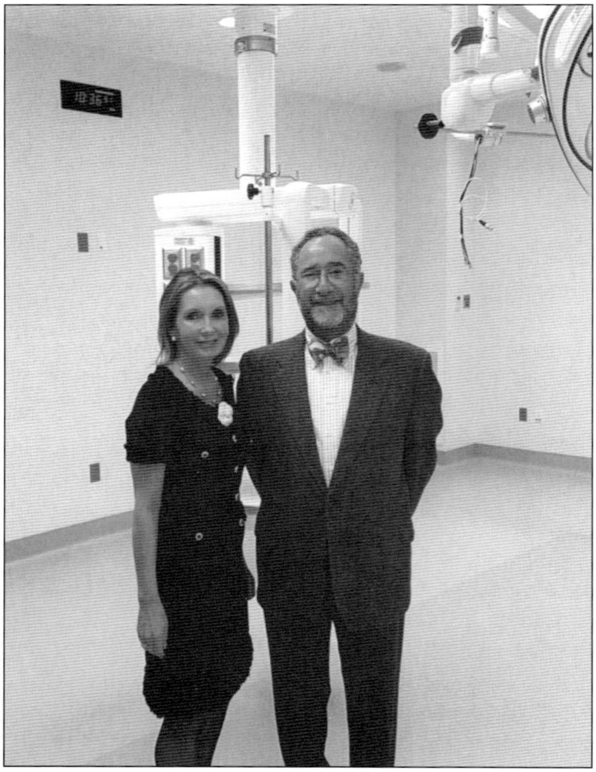

Mary and Rob Cohn, co-chairs of the surgery building fundraising drive, are shown in a nearly completed operating room in April 2016. The white structure behind them is a ceiling-mounted boom that replaces the need for cables or hoses underfoot for electricity, medical gases, and suction. In the Russell Surgery Building, completed in 1975, the operating rooms ranged in size from 350 square feet to 550 square feet, while the new building to open in June 2016 will range from 550 square feet up to 750 square feet. (Photograph by Kelli Rafferty.)

The new surgical building nears completion in 2016. When operational, it will provide state-of-the-art facilities for contemporary surgery. The ground floor includes an entry lobby, mechanical support, and shell space for future expansion. (Photograph by Daren Gray.)

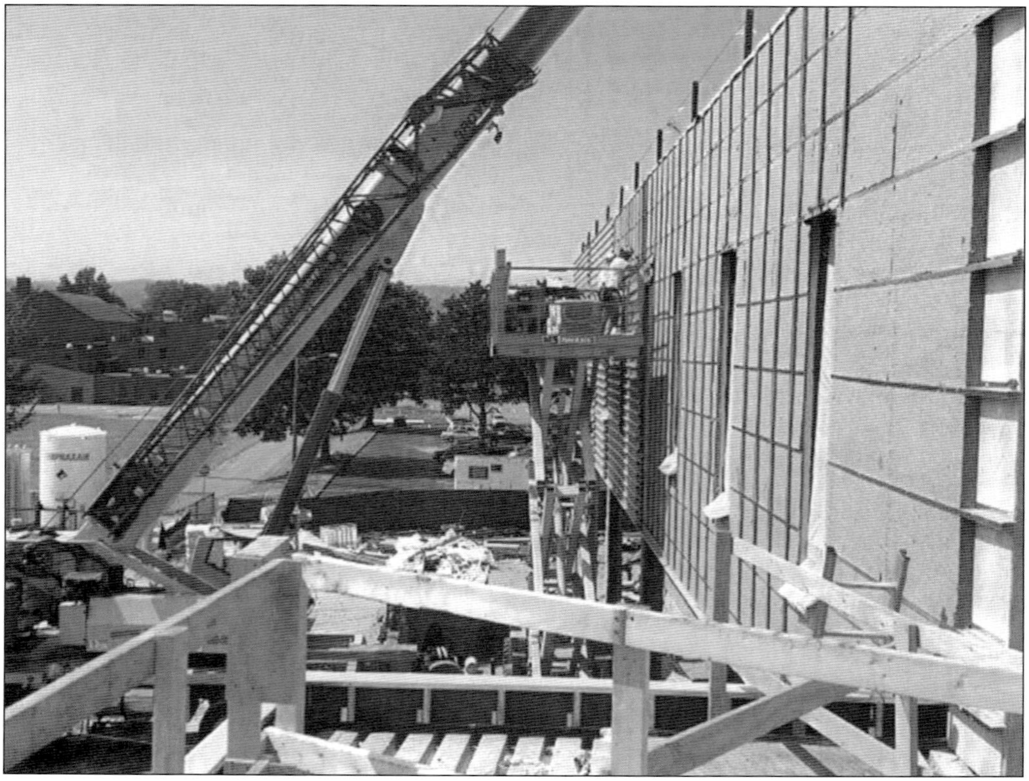

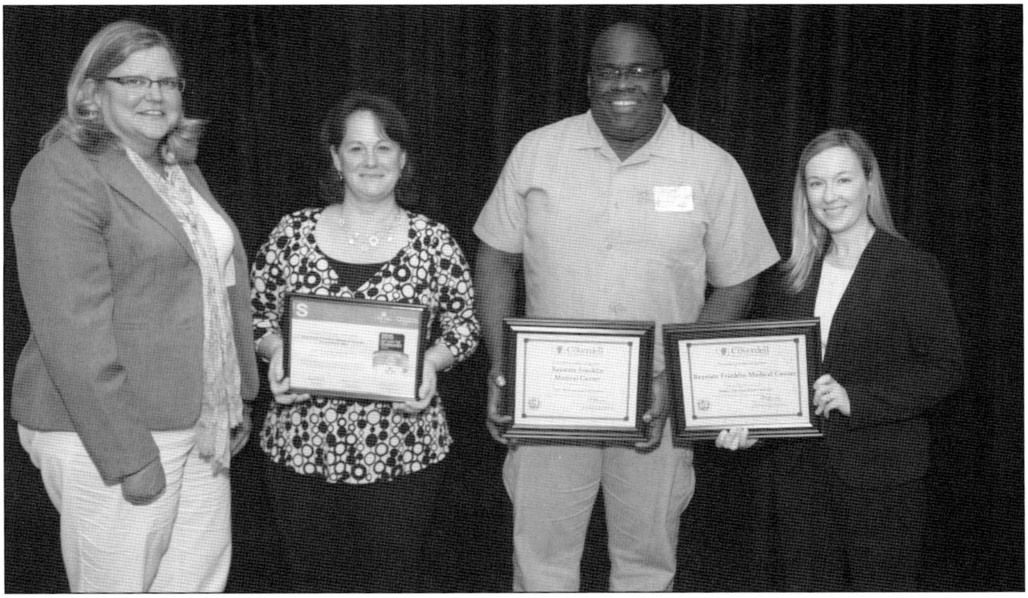

BFMC's campaign to keep care local has resulted in award-winning care for heart attack and stroke patients through telemedicine-guided treatment. In 2015, Diane Stephan, RN (Emergency Department nurse educator), and Charles Redd, RN (Emergency Department manager), accepted awards from Lea Susan Ojamaa (far left) of the Massachusetts Department of Public Health and Lisa Bemben (far right) of the Massachusetts and Rhode Island American Heart Association/American Stroke Association.

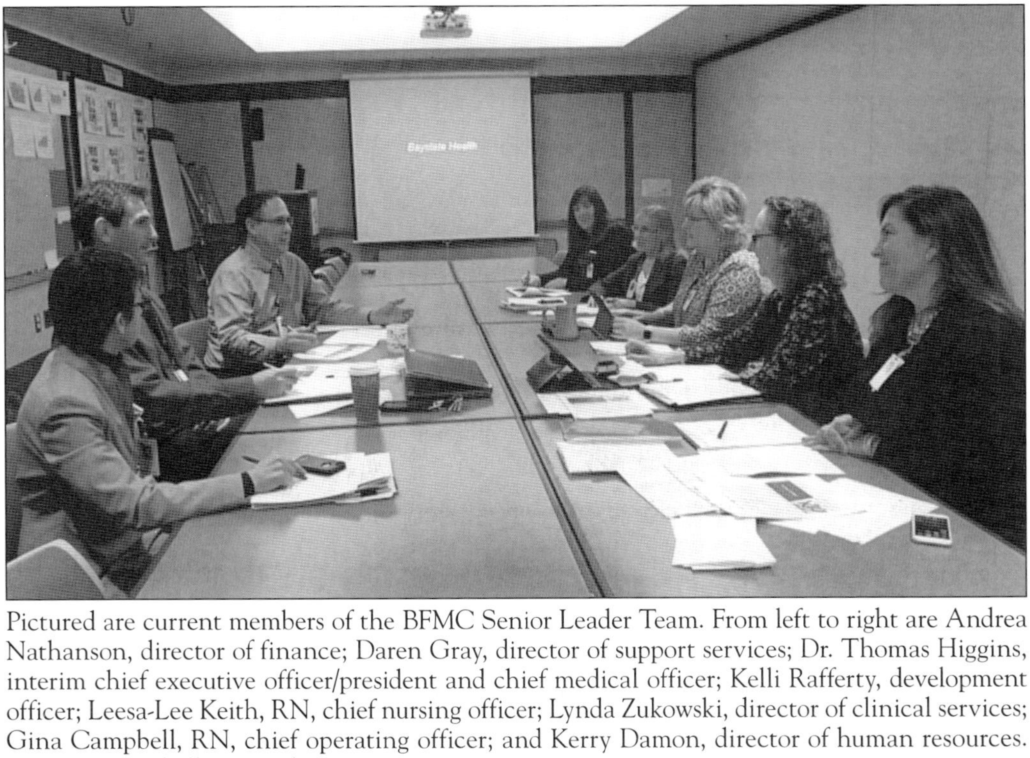

Pictured are current members of the BFMC Senior Leader Team. From left to right are Andrea Nathanson, director of finance; Daren Gray, director of support services; Dr. Thomas Higgins, interim chief executive officer/president and chief medical officer; Kelli Rafferty, development officer; Leesa-Lee Keith, RN, chief nursing officer; Lynda Zukowski, director of clinical services; Gina Campbell, RN, chief operating officer; and Kerry Damon, director of human resources. (Courtesy of Phyllis Stone.)

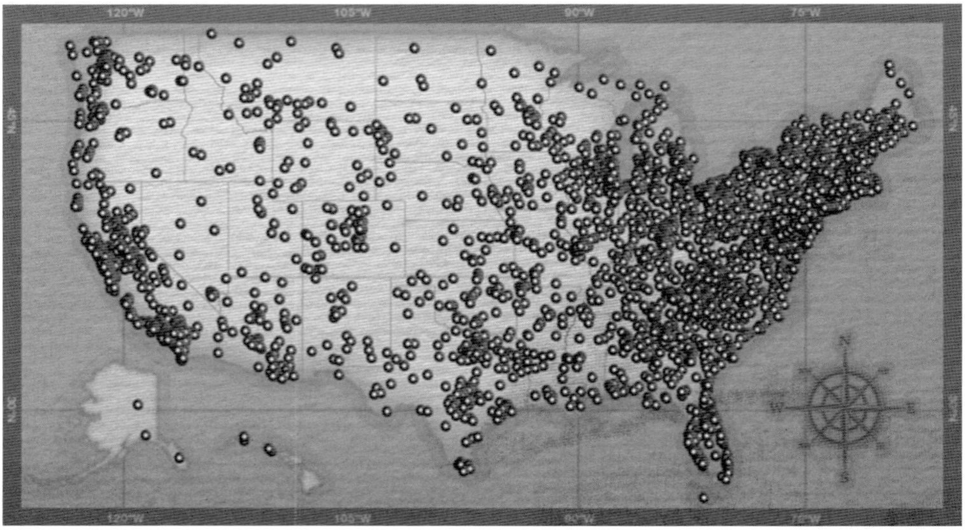